ASIAN *beauty* SECRETS

ANCIENT AND MODERN TIPS FROM THE FAR EAST

MARIE JHIN, M.D.

Asian Beauty Secrets:
Ancient and Modern Tips from the Far East

ISBN: 9780615405353
Library of Congress Control Number: 2011928662

Bush Street Press
237 Kearny Street, #174
San Francisco, CA 94108
415-413-0785

Cover Design by Zoe Lonergan, zoelonergan@gmail.com

Photo of Marie Jhin courtesy of Richard Martinez, dollyphotos@gmail.com

The information provided in this book is designed to provide helpful information on the subjects discussed. This book is not meant to be used, nor should it be used, to diagnose or treat any medical condition. For diagnosis or treatment of any medical problem, consult your own physician. The publisher and author are not responsible for any specific health or allergy needs that may require medical supervision and are not liable for any damages or negative consequences from any treatment, action, application, or preparation to any person reading or following the information in this book. References are provided for informational purposes only and do not constitute endorsement of any websites or other sources. Readers should be aware that the Web sites listed in this book may change.

Printed in the United States of America

ENDORSEMENTS

Having beautiful skin is the eternal pursuit for most people. Dr. Jhin's "Asian Beauty Secrets" helps us uncover those secrets for eternal beauty and health from Asia. From her extensive research and in depth and extensive knowledge of these Asian products, she lets us know that beautiful skin has no age limits.
- Liu Na, Host, Hunan Satellite TV, "Encyclopedia said"

Ancient Asian Beauty is simple, reasonable, and natural. It includes the concept of the whole, which includes internal and external beauty. The book informs us that beauty is self-cultivated, from the inside out. The book also stresses the importance of cultivating a lifestyle where one's own unique beauty is important.   - Zhuang Yan, Shanghai TV Host

I refuse to blindly use cosmetic products, but I would rather understand the real needs of the skin. Dr. Jhin's book, Asian Beauty Secrets, explains the origins of Asian skin care. It is like a skin care bible that reasonably teaches us the secrets of the skin and how to best take care of it.   - Dai Yue, the 1st "Super Idol" Competition, China

I like the simple skin care regimen that is natural and delicate. Since I grew up in the highlands, I have respect for nature. I feel that Dr. Jhin's book, Asian Beauty Secrets, reveals and outlines those natural secrets of Ancient Asia from Japan, Korea, and China that were used for the skin, as well as her professional recommendations.
-Yang Xiucuo, Super Idol, Blossoming Flowers Contest, China

In Asian Beauty Secrets, Dr. Marie Jhin draws on her experience as a dermatologist and combines this with her knowledge of Asian beauty remedies, both ancient and modern. The result? A wonderful East-West guide to vibrant skin.
- Jill Blakeway, M.Sc., L.Ac. and Founder of The YinOva Center

As a fifth-generation Asian-American, I'm delighted that Dr. Jhin has created our definitive guide to the secrets of beautiful, healthful, radiant skin. All that, of course, plus an ever-renewing prescription for plenty of good sex.

- Dr. Sadie Allison, Bestselling Author, *Ride 'Em Cowgirl! Sex Position Secrets for Better Bucking*

What a fascinating and enlightening book Dr. Jhin has given us. Asian Beauty Secrets reveals why centuries-old customs have withstood the test of time; it explains how nurturing inner beauty enhances outer beauty, and it offers sensible, <u>natural</u> approaches to achieving the beauty of the ages—Asian beauty. There is nothing radical here, just some of the most effective—and sometimes surprising—beauty tips you will ever find.

- Spencer Christian, Weatherman/Host ABC TV

Asian Beauty Secrets by Dr. Jhin reveals concepts and beauty treatments that are not only unique, but also easily attainable. I love the Korean concept of "outer radiance depends on inner harmony." As a dermatologist, I am also impressed by her real skin solution treatments and trends. This is truly a "beautiful" book!

- Debra B. Luftman, M.D., Beverly Hills Dermatologist and Co-Author of *The Beauty Prescription*

Dr. Jhin shows us the importance of maintaining our health and beauty through the use of centuries-old and well-tested ways. It is clear that old wives' tales are really the secrets for long-term, overall thriving, best achieved though the gentle treatment of our bodies. We learn that nature has the support we need, and Dr. Jhin's storytelling reveals how to use it. I love how she brings us to nature.

- Elisabeth Thieriot, Founder of LionsGateLiving.com and Author of *Be Fabulous at Any Age*

This book is dedicated to:

My parents, who have always been my biggest fans and who continue to want the best for me;

My kids, Cairo, Cooper, and Kylie, whom I love very much and inspire me every day to laugh, be inquisitive, and never give up;

and

Lance, for being my partner and support in this adventurous ride through life.

Love you all!

CONTENTS

Introduction

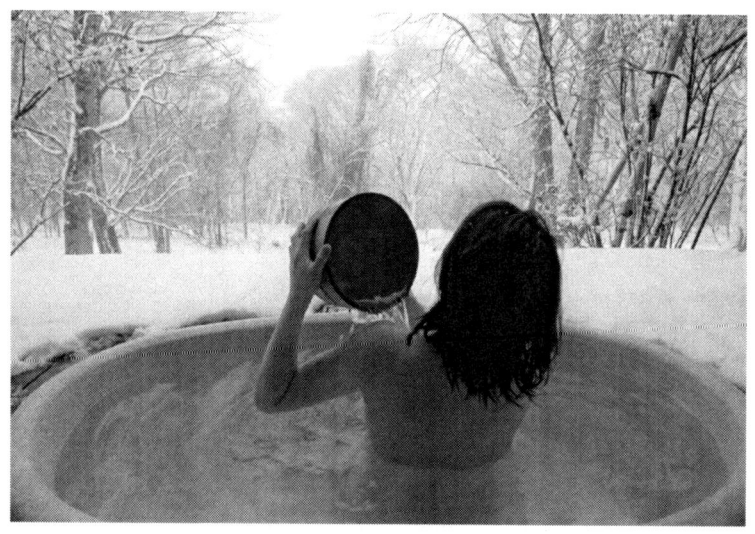

INTRODUCTION

A S A SAN FRANCISCO board-certified dermatologist, I've always been fascinated by beauty "secrets" of women from the Far East. This fascination is especially significant since I was born in Seoul, South Korea.

I have fond memories of going to communal Korean women's baths with my grandmother, mom, and aunts. We would spend a few hours bathing and exfoliating our skin with scrub towels. Like the other women, we emerged clean, purified in body and senses, and totally refreshed and rejuvenated with new energy. When I came to the United States, I continued with my past bathing and skin exfoliation regimens.

I also remember that my mom worried I looked tired and pale from working too hard as a medical student at Cornell University. She gave me *han yak,* or Chinese herbal medicine, to drink. I didn't argue with my mother and took the concoctions as directed, even though I wasn't sure what ingredients were in them. I had to heat and drink them every night, but I remember they were not tasty and that I did not enjoy them!

When I had my three children, my mother again presented me with her traditional advice and folklore. She told me that after a pregnancy, it was very important for the body to stay warm—especially during the first month. This philosophy is very different from mothers in this country who are out and about, strolling with their new babies as soon as they possibly can. I tried to stay indoors and kept my babies indoors, too.

When I had to go outside, my mom made me cover my head with a scarf. And after each pregnancy, my mother diligently prepared seaweed soup for me to drink—every day. She told me it would keep my body warm and help me produce abundant milk. Again, I didn't argue and did what she advised. Sure enough, I had more than enough breast milk.

These traditions and folklore have continued to fascinate me as an adult and, more important, as a doctor and dermatologist. As a scientist who regularly gives out prescription remedies or recommends beauty products, I make sure there is some science behind most of the beauty products I recommend—ideally based on double-blind studies, with placebo-controlled clinical data.

I share this to provide some explanation as to why my cultural background and professional curiosity make me *want* to answer some of my longstanding questions. What are these "ancient secrets" or traditions for health and beauty? What is the history or folklore about them? Is there any science to back them up? Why do women and men in Asia, as well as those in this country who have Asian backgrounds, continue using some of these centuries-old traditions?

Asians are often thought by many to have beautiful skin. Is it all genetics, or are there "secrets" we can learn from various Chinese, Korean, and Japanese treatments and traditions? While we may never know all of the answers to our satisfaction, it is for the purpose of seeking the truth that I was prompted to write this book. I hope the summary of my findings is of benefit to you, even as it helps me answer these questions.

As a dermatologist, I recognize that not all skin types are alike. Even within the Asian community, there are many shades and variations. I have chosen Japan, Korea, and China because in my practice, I have found them to share similar skin issues and concerns. I will present these issues in later chapters.

Moreover, due to a heightened interest today in the emergence of Asia and Asian cultures as innovative and growing a commanding marketing presence around the world, I would also like to discuss modern and popular treatments, along with some non-conventional ones that are currently being pursued by Asians in Asia.

My vision and goals in writing this book are to discover:

1. Ancient Asian beauty and skin care secrets from Korea, Japan, and China;

2. How relevant these beauty "secrets" are today;

3. How east-west perceptions of beauty dovetail and diverge;

4. How modern women are re-fashioning these ancient secrets into practical beauty and skin care applications to feel and look their best today;

5. How Far East Asian skin is different and what some common issues are;

6. What current treatments are available, and how popular and appropriate these are.

However, let me also point out that these are centuries-old "secrets" passed down through generations. I'm listing them without making any value judgments. I'm also not seeking or offering scientific validation for why and how they came about. It's my hope that you enjoy an Asian beauty tour with these intriguing stories. Adapt them as you like—many "secrets" become apparent as to why they originated when we understand their healing and medicinal properties as explained by modern science.

RESEARCH METHODOLOGY

My research method includes:

- Interviews with more traditional Asian medicine practitioners, such as acupuncturists and herbal medicine doctors.

- Email inquiries and surveys to friends and colleagues for Asian beauty and health secrets.
- Email interviews with overseas experts.
- Online research.
- Library research.

WHAT IS BEAUTY?

As the saying goes, "Beauty is in the eye of the beholder." What does this mean?

It means there are various ways of looking attractive, and *how* different cultures see beauty varies, as well. However, the overriding goal in every culture is for a person to present an attractive appearance—starting from the top on down, for a polished presentation that generates confidence in the eye of the beholder.

Upon meeting someone, you first notice the face, followed by the hair, which invariably places more emphasis on the head and shoulders and how the glowing radiance of a friendly, smiling face is a statement of true beauty in itself. Thus, many of these ancient secrets focus on facial skin and hair and continue to excite and invigorate the imagination of today's women in "looking lovely."

It's fascinating how many unique Asian beauty and skin care methods have withstood the test of time and are still being used in their original forms—such as nightingale poop for a geisha-style facial. Even more amazing is that there are women paying $180 for a 60-minute session at Shizuka New York Day Spa. (That's before tax and gratuity.)[1]

On their website, Shizuka explains how *uguisu no fun* ('no fun?'), or powdered nightingale bird droppings, saved the lives of geishas and Kabuki theater actors who faced chronic skin conditions from using makeup laced with zinc and lead.

---

[1] http://www.shizukany.com/geisha-facial.htm

Today, as the National Human Genome Research Institute explains, guanine is one of four integral parts making up the body's DNA.[2] That's why, although they may appear as lowly droppings on the surface, nightingale guanine speeds up skin healing on an esteemed level.

A celebrity who had to use foundation to hide blemishes thrives on Shizuka's geisha facial. *The Telegraph* reported that for the first time in years, former Spice Girl "Posh"-turned-fashion-designer Victoria Beckham[3] has smooth and supple skin. The droppings are mixed with rice bran and water to make the facial mask. (BTW, rice bran water is another nature-based facial cleanser Asian women use.)

That's also how this sweet songbird has come to symbolize beauty in Japan, too.

ASIAN BEAUTY SECRETS ARE ROOTED IN NATURE

Japanese women are noted for their doll-like, fine porcelain skin. As reported by Britain's *The Telegraph* in this same October 16, 2008 article, Victoria Beckham found her "latest beauty secret" when she visited Japan.

Telegraph reporter Melissa Whitworth had to try it for herself. Her findings? "It produces the same results as a light acid peel, but it causes none of the redness or the need for recovery time. There's no burning sensation and no man-made chemicals. Because of this, the geisha facial can be done on the day of a red-carpet appearance or an important party. It's also safe for pregnant women."

Ms. Whitworth concludes: "I have to admit that my skin looks extraordinarily healthy and bright. My squeamishness was banished after smelling the inoffensive powder and

---

[2] http://www.genome.gov/glossary/?id=96
[3] http://fashion.telegraph.co.uk/article/TMG3365670/Geisha-facial-the-latest-beauty-secret-of-Victoria-Beckham-brought-to-the-masses.html

realizing it had been finely milled, cleaned, and sterilized" by UV (ultra-violet light)—without even a chance of catching avian flu.

One of my dermatology medical assistants is Chinese. Her mother shared some beauty secrets from China. These, too, are animal- and nature-based, thus reinforcing how systemic and interconnected our natural world is—among humans, animals, plants, the universe, and the universal energy or life force, *qi.*

Take for instance, "Hasma snow frog." Jacqueline M. Newman[4] was at a lucky spot in China while searching for the origins of this exotic animal. She found it's also called forest, grass, or white frogs (because of their white underbellies). Caught before or during the first snowfall just before hibernation, snow frogs are richly fortified with hormones and high in lipids—before these female frogs lay oodles of eggs come spring. It's little wonder that snow frogs are highly prized for moisturizing and reviving body cells by Chinese women.

You'll find the recipe for Hasma snow frog soup in Chapter 4, where we discuss more amazing beauty rituals originating in ancient China.

As we're aware, skin needs to be moisturized to maintain smoothness, clarity, and suppleness. This is an important aspect that impacts overall body health. We recognize that true beauty wells up from deep within and is much more than the sum of outer appearances. By nourishing and moisturizing body cells on a deeper level, from the inside out, a person's health is clearly reflected on the body's largest organ—the skin and the face.

Another Chinese beauty *and* health secret is swallow's nest. Three times a year, swallows build their nests in caves—only to be robbed of them by beauty booty hunters. This multi-million dollar industry started during China's Tang

---

[4] http://www.flavorandfortune.com/dataaccess/article.php?ID=248

Dynasty (618-907). It was first mentioned in Gu Ming's *Guidelines on Diet* during the Yuan Dynasty (around 1350). Clearly, this was and still is a culinary delicacy prized by wealthy Chinese.

Biochemists C. Y. Kong and P. S. Kwan[5] of Chinese Hong Kong University report swallow's nests are made from the birds' saliva and imbued with water-soluble protein. Rich in amino acids that proteins need to build body cells, swallow's nest improves skin tone, balances qi (or life force energy), aids in respiratory ailments, and enhances immunity. We have a fun recipe to try out in Chapter 4.

TWO ANCIENT ASIAN NATURE BEAUTY SECRETS:

1. Nightingale poop helps skin recover from acne and other blemishes.
2. Swallow's nests tone skin and regenerate body cells.

We'll be discussing lots more ancient Asian beauty secrets based on Mother Nature's healing gifts.

ASIAN BEAUTY SECRETS ARE ROOTED IN GOOD FOOD

It's clear by now how very elemental Asian beauty secrets are in depending on healing foods from the plant and animal kingdoms. However, it bears pointing out that food-based healing is also universal. Greek physician Hippocrates (460-377 BCE), "the father of modern medicine," was unequivocal about the healing power of food and its impact on the body's systemic functions.

---

[5] http://www.e2121.com/food_db/viewherb.php3?viewid=214&setlang

In Korea, and now renowned worldwide, ginseng is the wonder tonic for whole body healing and metabolic exchanges by helping food digest properly.[6] Essential nutrients become more easily absorbed, instead of being eliminated. Just as incredible, ginseng juice is great as a shampoo; it also volumizes, detangles, and moisturizes—to bestow a healthy crown of lustrous hair.

In Japan, wakame seaweed is big time. Rich in essential minerals and vitamins, this superfood's outstanding contribution to healthy skin is a wealth of hyaluronic acid that's vital in helping skin retain the moisture it needs. With over 70 percent of the body consisting of water, hyaluronic acid is imperative in plumping up skin to look healthy, toned, firm, and vibrant with good health.

TWO ANCIENT ASIAN FOOD BEAUTY SECRETS:

1. Ginseng is an incredible skin and overall body tonic.
2. Seaweed nourishes body cells while moisturizing skin.

ASIAN BEAUTY SECRETS ARE ROOTED IN REBALANCING ENERGY

Feeling healthy in going with the flow translates into *wu-wei* for the Chinese. It means living effortlessly and graciously. Loosely translated as "right" natural action, westerners are more familiar with the yin-yang symbol enclosed within the circle of wu-wei. This elegant Daoist concept of natural living is an art form in itself to achieve.

Practitioners of Traditional Chinese Medicine (TCM) are experts when it comes to rebalancing energy so qi can flow along the body's energy meridians or pathways. When qi flows in tune with the body by adapting to the seasons, wu-wei enhances healing and dynamic living. That's where qi

[6] http://www.suite101.com/content/asian-beauty-secrets-a197245

gong and tai chi exercises (similar to hatha yoga) aid digestion, flexibility, suppleness, and body strength. Quietly passive, qi is, nevertheless, powerful, dynamic and restorative.Methods used in rebalancing energy more familiar to westerners include:

- Acupuncture. Practiced for over five thousand years in China, many prefer to go the route of needles instead of Botox®. After a diagnosis is made, fine, thin needles are inserted along meridians to unclog qi so healing can begin. This healing modality was introduced to Korea and Japan in the sixth century. In 1997, the U.S. National Institutes of Health (NIH) published a "Consensus Development Program," advising healthcare practitioners of acupuncture's efficacy.[7] We'll be discussing this in more detail later.

- Acupressure is less invasive than acupuncture. Pressure is applied either with appropriate massage or with cupping (wherein glass jars facilitate creating a vacuum) to unclog flows along energy meridians. Even Hippocrates used cupping to re-invigorate blood and lymph flows.[8]

TWO ANCIENT ASIAN ENERGY BEAUTY SECRETS:

1. Acupuncture is recognized by the National Institutes of Health (NIH) to be an effective medical intervention.
2. Acupressure is a non-invasive approach to reinvigorate energy flow.

ANCIENT ASIAN BEAUTY SECRETS AND TODAY'S LIFESTYLES

It's noteworthy how inviolable and universal beauty aspirations can be. For example:

---

[7] http://consensus.nih.gov/1997/1997Acupuncture107html.htm
[8] http://en.wikipedia.org/wiki/Fire_cupping

- <u>Quest to be liked and trusted.</u> *Time Asia*'s poignant article on how plastic surgery helps job-seekers in Asia regain personal esteem by going under the knife is a reminder of why beauty is only skin deep.[9]

- <u>Quest to look more western.</u> Double-eyelid surgery (blepharoplasty) among Asians in the U.S. is becoming more popular, notes Bruce Cunningham, M.D. and past president of the American Society of Plastic Surgeons.[10] It's also highly popular in Korea, Japan, and China.

- <u>Quest to look more refined with lighter skin.</u> It's an ingrained cultural desire among upper-class women in the Far East to look fairer and whiter. This is evident in the use of umbrellas to avoid sun damage to the skin. However, many are in it only for the looks.

I conclude this introduction by mentioning a treatment for the "sweet spot." The *Los Angeles Times* (12/20/2010) article[11] on *chai-york* discusses the traditional Korean treatment for women. It's good for men's perineal parts, too. A centuries-old steaming method for the vagina to purge toxins, bladder infections, kidney problems, and infertility, it's a 14-herbal restorative tea pack, primarily laced with mugwort and wormwood. Mugwort is anti-bacterial, anti-fungal, and it rebalances women's hormones. Wormwood has anti-bacterial and anti-viral properties. There's more to come on chai-york as a spa treatment in Chapter 2.

Skeptics may call ancient health and beauty treatments an inaccurate science. But, as this book reveals, natural, herbal, and food remedies with healing pedigrees dating back centuries are compelling stories which are hard to ignore in the quest for beautiful skin and a healthy, happy lifestyle.

---

[9] http://www.time.com/time/asia/covers/1101020805/story4.html

[10] http://www.asian-nation.org/cosmetic-surgery.shtml

[11] http://articles.latimes.com/2010/dec/20/health/la-he-v-steam-20101220

Asian Beauty Secrets will give you time-tested traditions, natural remedies, and non-invasive enhancements to help you capture relevant beauty tips of the Far East that are easy to add or adapt to your current beauty regimen.

CHAPTER ONE

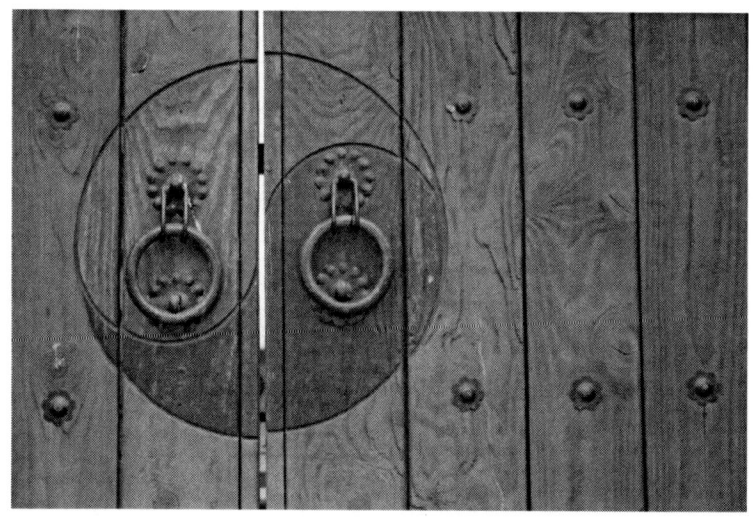

1

The History of Beauty
in the Far East

"Whiteness" or having white skin is considered an important element in constructing female beauty in Asian cultures. Not only does skin lightness affect perceptions of a woman's beauty, it also affects her marital prospects, job prospects, social status, and earning potential. The beauty ideal of white skin predates colonialism and the introduction of Western notions of beauty.
—Prof. Eric P.H. Li, York University, Canada; et. al.[12]

IMAGINE GETTING UP at the break of dawn to collect a few precious drops of fresh dew, then mixing this pure elixir of morning into a paste with delicate rose petal powder to apply on your cheeks so they blush naturally, like roses. It was for real and a traditional Korean beauty ritual all upper class women assiduously sought.

I find history so appealing—to show and teach later generations secrets and tips to experiment and adapt—in shining intriguing guidelines on innovations as necessitated by changing circumstances. We'll take a historical cultural beauty tour of Korea, Japan, and China in this chapter to find out what women in these countries did, and still do, in their quest to look beautiful.

---

[12] http://www.acrwebsite.org/volumes/v35/naacr_vol35_273.pdf

A HISTORY OF BEAUTY IN KOREA

To prove that Korean women in the 19th century (during the Joseon Dynasty) collected fresh dew for their beauty potions, the founder of a leading Korean cosmetics company has a museum dedicated to studying Korean beauty artifacts and rituals. Sang-ok Yoo has built Coréana cosmetics into a leading brand in his country.[13] Located in Seoul's Gangnam district, the Coréana Cosmetics Museum is a window of opportunity to peek into how Korean women in bygone eras nourished their skin and hair with the help of Mother Nature.

Mr. Yoo is quoted in a *Joong Ang* newspaper (11/29/2004) article as knowledgeable on how young women of Korea's 6th century Silla Dynasty cared for their skin and hair—such as massaging peony flower oil into the scalp to produce a shining mane. (You may have also watched the Korean TV mini-series on Queen Son Deuk, a Silla ruler who was a mighty warrior at that time.)

Korean women had an innate wisdom in concocting beauty treatments. After hundreds of years, this museum's collection of small vanity glass items—two-inch wide potion bottles, jars, and dishes—are still crystal clear and clean. Mr. Yoo explained, "Joseon women used all natural things, which don't stain."

Korean women are reputed to have the fairest Far Eastern Asian skin. This understanding of how nature's elemental forces and energies can work to their advantage by using women's beauty secrets is astutely harnessed by Korean cosmetics companies.

In its major U.S. launch in summer 2010, Korean cosmetics company Amore Pacific introduced their "Sulwhasoo" line to New York City's top beauty emporium—Bergdorf Goodman.[14] On its website, Bergdorf

---

[13] http://www.inescho.com/articlepdf/041509062435.pdf
[14] http://blog.bergdorfgoodman.com/womens-style/sulwhasoo

Goodman explains the basic tenet of Korean beauty: *"Outer radiance depends on inner harmony."* Radiance is further defined as a natural glow that's not greasy looking.

Bergdorf Goodman explains Korean herbal medicine knows the body undergoes internal changes every seven years. Along with these changes, the skin becomes dull, loses its elasticity and firmness, and thins out. In the past, this major shift would be noticed around a person's 35th year.

However, with the hectic pace of living today, combined with environmental pollutants and excess stress in meeting deadlines, the body loses its internal balance even earlier. Since the body works in synchronicity with all its parts and reacts systemically, this imbalance also impacts skin by reducing vital energy that's needed to produce and maintain clear, elastic, and well-toned skin.

Enter ginseng, a highly-revered herbal adaptogen with the ability to restore and rebalance the body's natural healing energies. Korean ginseng is world-renowned as the best in the world.

As referenced on Bergdorf Goodman's website, Korean medical concepts are based on the 25-volume *Donguibogam* or "Principles and Practice of Eastern Medicine," codified by Heo Jun in 1610 and recognized by royal decree in 1613.[15] Additionally, this era's progressive thinking also started an innovative public health system to benefit everyone. Emphasis was placed on prevention, rather than medical intervention. The UNESCO document cited by Bergdorf Goodman's Web site calls this health care philosophy significant, important, and incomparable to anything else in the world at that time (even as its benefits are felt today).

As a leading-edge authority on natural Korean medical herbal and energy doctrines, this philosophy provides a well-informed code for women's cosmetics. Bergdorf Goodman

---

15

http://portal.unesco.org/ci/en/files/27075/12133693253Korea_Donguib ogam.pdf/Korea%2BDonguibogam.pdf says they haven't seen any skin care treatment like Sulwhasoo's that's entirely herbal-based—with an ounce of Concentrated Ginseng Cream selling for $220—and women gladly shell out for it.

Analogous to the Chinese doctrine of yin-yang, the Korean *sang seng* principle recognizes the need to re-balance the body's opposing energies into a harmonious whole. That's why you feel great after a soothing massage, relaxing bath, or facial—when physical energy is naturally re-balanced, re-centered, and harmonized internally with emotional, mental, vital, and spiritual energies.

Jill Blakeway, founder and CEO of YinOva Center in New York City, explains the composition of Sulwhasoo Concentrated Ginseng Cream according to yin-yang principles.[16] Qi and yang energy are found in tonics, such as ginger and astragalus—which reduce puffiness under the eyes, tone the skin by making it more elastic, and improves blood circulation for a clearer complexion. Yin energy is found in the herbs rehmannia and ophiopogonis—which hydrate and moisturize skin at deeper levels, reduce inflammation to cool the skin, and nourish skin to reduce fine lines and wrinkles. Taken together, opposing energies are perfectly harnessed to complement skin wellness.

Another intriguing Korean beauty standard is striving for a lighter skin and flawless complexion. While contemporary reasoning may attribute this beauty standard to present-day westernization, Prof. Eric P.H. Li of York University in Canada presents earlier findings to support the case for lightening skin. "In Korea, flawless skin like white jade and an absence of freckles and scars have been preferred since the first dynasty in Korean history (the *Gojoseon Era*, 2333-108 B.C.E.). Various methods of lightening the skin have long been used in Korea, such as applying *miansoo* lotion and dregs of honey."[17]

---

[16] http://www.yinovacenter.com/blog/archives/5677/
[17] http://www.acrwebsite.org/volumes/v35/naacr_vol35_273.pdf

Prof. Li and his co-authors explain it's deeply ingrained across cultures for shades of white to connote purity, chastity, righteousness, decency, and auspiciousness; while black or darker skin color infers less than preferred attributes of villainy, wickedness, and menace. Their article in *Advance in Consumer Research* (Volume 35, 2008) concludes with this dictum: Presenting whiteness in a person is preferred as it connotes prestige and a luxurious life, not just in Asia, but also worldwide.

However, there is a rash of western beauty fads at work in Korea today—for double eyelid surgery or blepharoplasty. An online source purportedly cites $1,100 for this surgery in South Korea—compared to $4,600 in the U.S.[18]

According to the International Society of Aesthetic Plastic Surgery figures for 2009 (latest available as of February, 2011), South Korea has emerged as the country with the highest per capita rate to go under the knife for cosmetic reasons—securing jobs and increasing earning potential and marital chances.[19] Blepharoplasty (double eyelid surgery) and rhinoplasty (nose jobs) are so common in Seoul's Apgujeong district that anyone can find these stops handily labeled on subway maps.[20]

We have lots more to chew on in the next chapter on what's brewing in Korea.

A HISTORY OF BEAUTY IN JAPAN

Continuing with the Far Eastern beauty standard of preferring a lighter shade of white skin, Prof. Eric Li and his colleagues found the reason for this preference among

---

[18] http://www.articleshub.org/article/2545/Plastic-Surgery-Holds-Key-to-South-Koreas-Medical-Tourism-Growth.html
[19] http://www.asianplasticsurgeryguide.com/news10-2/081003_south-korea-highest.html
[20] http://www.psfk.com/2010/08/enovate-chinese-youth-create-new-standards-of-beauty-online.html

Japanese women was to blend in with social norms. In other words, they didn't whiten their skin to enhance appearances. Rather, the Japanese saw whiteness to be all about social identity—and one that's even superior to Western whiteness.[21]

Culturally, Japanese men preferred their women *mochihada*, or "skin like pounded rice." Since the peaceful and prosperous Edo Dynasty (1603-1867), Japanese women have considered it "a moral duty" to apply white powder on their faces since their beauty was judged according to this decree.

Today, more than 90 percent of Japanese women adopt this beauty code in public, this same research paper states.[22] Even modern-day tanning aficionadas honor this standard by preserving and presenting flawlessly whitened faces.

How do Japanese women maintain their flawless complexion? We've explained the science behind nightingale guano facials. Other techniques include:

- Pitera, a fermenting yeast. England's *Daily Mail* newspaper (June 25, 2007) reports top model Kate Moss uses the Japanese whitening agent pitera that's derived from sake.[23] The legend goes that an observant monk found a Kobe monastery renowned for distilling sake, or rice wine, had monks whose hands were softer, suppler, smoother, and more youthful looking. Before long, pitera's nutrients became the rage for Japanese skin care manufacturers, such as Shiseido, in forging a worldwide cult following.

- *Onsen* hot springs. Laced with minerals, Japan's naturally occurring onsen or hot springs are gorgeous spas set amidst spectacular volcanic scenery. Men and women think nothing of stepping into the healing

---

[21] http://www.acrwebsite.org/volumes/v35/naacr_vol35_273.pdf
[22] Ibid.
[23] http://www.dailymail.co.uk/femail/article-464194/Turning-Japanese-beauty-thats-taking-over.html

waters—in the buff, save for a dainty towel over the head.

- *Sento* hot baths. Communal bathing (unisex or gender separate) relaxes body-mind-spirit. However, proper etiquette requires a total scrub down first, before entering *all* baths. Taking hot baths improves the body's circulation while increasing its metabolism, so body cells are revived with more oxygen and toxins are disposed of—with skin becoming revitalized and robust looking.

- Collagen. Collagen keeps skin soft, firm, smooth, and youthful looking. Oprah reported on her TV show that Japanese women mix powdered collagen (from pigs, chickens, cows, and fish) with water to drink. It's a daily ritual for the skin. However, it does not work on erasing wrinkles. You can watch the video of this show by visiting www.oprah.com/style/Japanese-Beauty-Secrets-Video.

  The question might be asked: why inject botox when you can eat and drink collagen for overall body health? A person would also be less likely to suffer facial redness, discomfort, and bruising.

- Camellia oil or *tsubaki.* The flower that signals early spring gifts Japanese women in wondrous other ways. Camellia oil promotes hair growth, leaving it soft, manageable, not weighted down, nor greasy looking. It's also great for fading stretch marks and acne scars, while helping oily skin re-moisturize naturally by not clogging the pores. Camellia oil also softens cuticles and is reported to be terrific for treating burns. How can one not love this oil?

  Source:
  http://www.iheartdaily.com/2009/11/japanese-beauty-secret-camellia-oil.html

- <u>Seaweed.</u> In this book's introduction, I mentioned the moisturizing benefits of hyaluronic acid found in wakame seaweed. Another wonderful seaweed is nori—the tasty seaweed that's wrapped around sushi. Nori is great for glossy, healthy hair because of iodine (not iodine added to table salt, which the body doesn't absorb easily.) Iodine nourishes hair, along with traces of iron, zinc, selenium, and copper that are found in nori seaweed.

Lustrous long hair has always been a beauty standard across cultures. In Japan, dating as far back as the Heian Dynasty (734-1185), women of the Imperial Court showed off long tresses, with the record at 23-feet long.[24] Beauty was further enhanced with heavy white rice powder for faces and necks, red pouty lips, narrow eyes, thin noses, and blackened teeth with charcoal to match the hair.

As these examples show, the art of Japanese beauty was, and still is, derived from Mother Nature. Today, such beautiful gifts are admired and used globally—thanks to Japanese cosmetics companies such as Shiseido and Kanebo.

A HISTORY OF BEAUTY IN CHINA

It's been said that diamonds are a girl's best friend. However, in ancient China, pearls were a woman's best friend when it came to maintaining her beauty with a flawless, lustrous skin. Today, pearls are *still* a beauty secret beloved by Chinese and Indian women. Ancient Egyptian and Mayan women knew the powerful effects of taking pearl powder, too.

Ground pearl powder was taken internally and applied topically by the likes of Empress Wu Ze Tian, who lived from 625-705 A.C.E. When she ascended the throne at 65, her

---

[24] http://asianhistory.about.com/od/japan/a/HeianBeauty.htm

legendary beauty cast a youthful radiance that women envied.[25] Of course, only the very best real pearl nacre was reserved for the Imperial family. Lesser grade pearl powder was crushed from mother-of-pearl and oyster shell. Worse, chalk could be added as fillers.

Why is pearl powder such a big beauty deal? Here are some reasons as explained by modern science. According to French scientists at the Museum D'Histoire de Naturelle's Biophysics Laboratory in Paris, pearl nacre is key in regenerating collagen.[26] Their research showed pearl nacre produces:

- Anti-aging effects, such as reducing wrinkles and age or sunspots.
- Collagen after the body stops producing it around age 40.
- Collagen renewal in bones and bone density, as well.
- A powerful anti-oxidant effect in slowing down cell disintegration.
- Healing by soothing inflammation, and it is especially good for sensitive skin in reducing redness and other skin irritations.
- Overall optimal health for the body, including enhancing eyesight.

Another favorite of Chinese royalty was jade. Empress Cixi was reported to have used a pure jade roller to massage her facial muscles.[27] Regular massage helps the lymphatic system flush out metabolic wastes, instead of letting toxins accumulate—which produces a puffy-looking face.

---

[25] http://www.whiterskin.info/the-use-of-pearl-powder-for-beautiful-youthful-skin-through-the-ages/

[26] http://extranet.securefreedom.com/PearlciumInternational/Personal/Resources/pearlcium%20product-Scientific%20Research-edited.doc

[27] http://www.study-in-china.org/ChinaFeature/Custom/2009510201764605.htm

This same article also cites the most famous concubine in Chinese history, Yang Yuhuan, in using litchi fruit and luxuriating in hot spring baths to nourish her delicate and ravishing skin. Daoist empress Wu Zeitan, true to her inner wisdom, took time out to close her eyes, tune out distracting thoughts, and revitalize her body and spirit with down time; and she successfully appeared rejuvenated. Today, we know how vital rest and a sound sleep are in sustaining—"a beauty rest."

And lest Chinese women forget, "A woman's second face is in her hands," as the saying goes. According to TCM (Traditional Chinese Medicine), the hands and feet represent microcosmic parts of the body. Jill Blakeway, founder of New York City's Yinova Center, explains her patients know to gently massage vital acu-points on their hands and feet to systemically impart an overall benefit of wellness to the body.[28]

Her suggestion? Simply looking after hands and feet pays dividends for health and beauty. Jill also notes how dark circles under the eyes call out for help to detoxify the kidneys. She prescribes reducing salt, swapping processed foods for nourishing whole foods, getting lots of sleep, and taking herbal adaptogen formulas.

Jill Blakeway highly recommends adaptogens from Nature's healing cupboard to help the body withstand stress while restoring balance. Such tonics include:

- reishi mushrooms to boost the immune system, help the liver regenerate, oxygenate blood, and re-balance blood sugar;
- schizandra is a powerful beauty tonic in preserving youthfulness by softening and moisturizing skin;
- astragalus rebalances body fluids, enhances immunity to diseases, and nurtures whole body living with more stamina.

---

[28] http://www.yinovacenter.com/blog/archives/1670/

Herbal remedies are age-old elixirs of life that have proven their worth through time. That's why Jill's first course of action for patients with skin problems is to purify the liver. She explains the liver cleanses impurities from the blood stream. However, a sluggish liver can't cleanse the blood properly of toxins—and enlists the skin to push out the "bad guys." That's how skin erupts with rashes and blemishes. The antidotes she suggests are: limiting alcohol and processed foods, plus taking liver-cleansing herbs, such as milk thistle, dandelion roots, and schizandra.

As Jill emphasizes in her beauty blog, TCM sees "beauty as a reflection of the state of someone's whole body. Radiance comes from a strong, vibrant spirit, good nourishment and enough rest. The holistic nature of Chinese medicine lends itself to the notion that beauty comes from within."[29]

While attempting to reach within for pearls of beauty to emerge, it's an ingrained cultural trait for Asians to take time out to enjoy life's more serene and slower moments, such as time for a meditative tea ceremony, a leisurely stroll in the park, releasing stress through tai chi or yoga, enjoying invigorating cups of white and green teas and ginseng tea, or just doing nothing—to rest and recharge the body's energy levels.

While it's true that Asian women don't have a peaches-and-cream complexion like Caucasian women do, it's highly plausible that the cool look of white jade and luxurious porcelain is a culturally ingrained goal in striving for whiteness by women of the Far East, and along with it, finding creative ways to lighten the skin.

In chapters to come, we explore skin issues faced by Asians of Korea, Japan, and China. We'll also cover what can be done to improve Asian skin conditions for men, women, and children.

---

[29] Ibid.

SOME JEWELS OF FAR EASTERN BEAUTY SECRETS

Korea:

- Outer beauty is a reflection of inner harmony.
- Beauty treatments are herbal-based, with many treatments using superior ginseng for satiny jade-like beauty.
- It has the world's highest per capita rates for going under the plastic knife—for blepharoplasty or double eyelid surgery.

Japan:

- Beauty treatments are nature-based—from taking collagen daily to nightingale guano facials for flawless skin.
- Purification of body and senses with water; sento and onsen baths are essential in maintaining a supple and smooth skin.
- Cultivating whiteness of skin is to manifest a strong socio-cultural identity.

China:

- TCM teaches beauty is not skin deep, but wells up from within in reflecting the body's total health and well-being.
- Recognizes that "a woman's second face is in her hands," and detoxifying the liver foremost to purify the blood—for beautiful skin.

My mother has beautiful, flawless-looking skin. I finally figured out her secret. Don't wear make-up! But as a TV broadcaster, I feel I have to wear foundation and powder because it makes my skin look better on air. The end result? Lots of clogged pores! Regular facials help, but my pores clog very quickly, even though I wash my face thoroughly every night.

However, on a recent extended vacation, I took a four-week break from wearing foundation. My pores cleared out completely within weeks. My friends noticed my skin looking smoother than ever. Now, I don't wear any foundation on air. I just dab a little concealer under the eyes and around the nose and use a kabuki brush to apply mineral powder all over my face. Now I have a TV-ready face, with lots less clogged-up pores. My skin may never look as good as my mom's, but it's certainly getting closer.

—Janelle Wang, San Francisco TV Broadcaster

Editorial Note: Mineral powder make-up consists of micronized titanium dioxide nano particles, which do not clog pores.

CHAPTER TWO

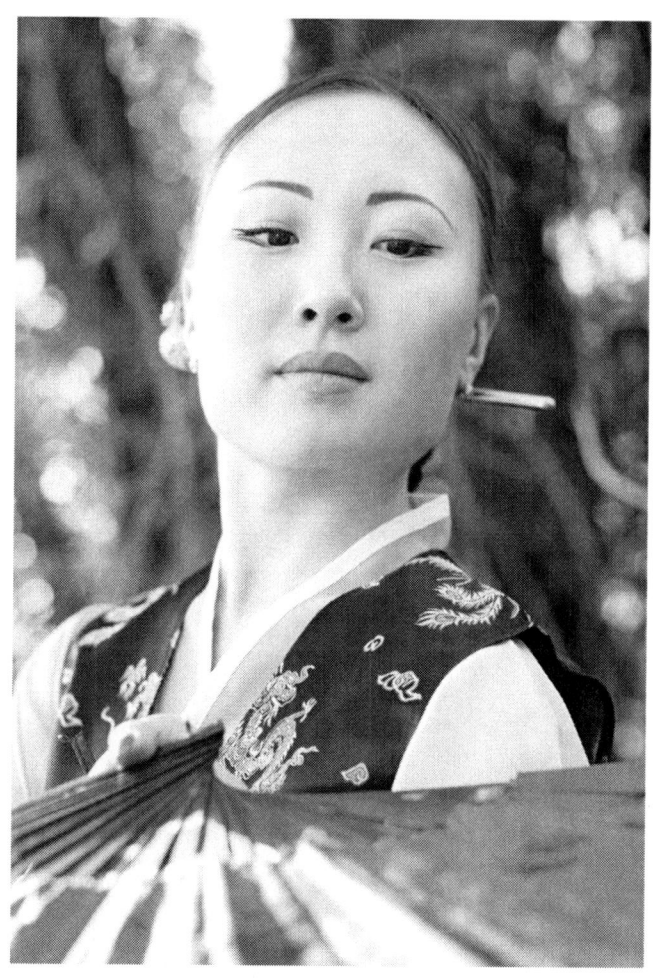

2

How is Beauty Defined in Korea?

The most popular procedure in Korea is the "double eyelid" operation to enlarge sleepy hooded eyes. Following a close second is the "nose job," which may or may not involve implanting a piece of silicone, gortex, or bone to heighten the bridge of the nose. Jaw shaving, which makes the traditionally wide Korean face smaller, used to be a popular, but dubious, procedure. These days, doctors are injecting botox into the jaw to make the muscle smaller, hence shrinking the face.

Youthful skin is also very important to Koreans, hence laser resurfacing, fat injections, peels, and botox are also high in demand. A new mini face-lift procedure called featherlift lifts saggy skin with tiny threads. With its low downtime, featherlift is fast becoming one of the most popular anti-aging procedures. Liposuction is done so often, even dermatologists and gynecologists are doing it as a 'lunchtime' procedure.

But, despite people's attempts to discount the importance of superficial beauty, there's just no denying that in Korea, as well as in most of the world, appearances and first impressions matter.   —SeoulStyle.com[30]

WHEN I WAS GROWING up in Seoul, South Korea, my grandma, mom, aunts, and I would take weekly baths together—not at home, but at Korean-style public baths—where we would spend a few hours "taking to the

---

[30] http://www.seoulstyle.com/art_plasticFantastic.htm

waters" amidst much laughter, fun, and harmless gossip, while strengthening our family ties even more.

I remember fondly having my body scrubbed clean. It was called *tae mi dah*, Korean for body scrub. My grandma and mother would tell me, "Come, scrub my back, because I cannot do it!" My eyes mist up as I recall my grandmother sitting on a small plastic stool, obviously enjoying her back scrub.

Tae means dirt in Korean, as in dirt or dead skin rolling off a person's back. Koreans love to exfoliate the skin to keep it glowing and healthy. Exfoliation is a cleansing process that scours and removes dead skin cells the body no longer needs. Skin cells renew and shed every 28 days, so they need to be cleaned off and washed away for both skin and body to stay healthy.

A Korean scrub is like getting a whole-body microdermabrasion in exfoliating the skin's top layer. This makes the skin smooth and helps promote cell turnover. A word of caution—aggressive scrubbing is especially irritating for sensitive skin.

That's why my female relatives and I would return home looking rosy-cheeked and vibrant with new energy—literally glowing in the pink of health. On a deeper level, we were emotionally nourished, as well, from the sense of community in renewing our friendships by taking communal baths together.

I left Korea when I was six for Hawaii, and eventually our family settled in New York City. There, I continued with my bathing and cleansing rituals at similar Korean-style saunas or bathhouses. And I still continue with it as an adult living in San Francisco.

Besides, it gives me time to de-stress and to rebalance physically and emotionally. Today, as a dermatologist with a full-time practice and the mother of three children, I enjoy taking monthly Korean-style baths, sitting in a hot steam room to unclog pores and to mindlessly bliss out—followed by a traditional scrub and massage.

(BTW, taking to the waters isn't only a Korean lifestyle practice. Asian and European cultures also "take to the waters" to maintain good health. The word "spa" is from the Latin healing concept, *salus per aquae*, or "health through water.")

That's why I'm very curious to find out what some of these ancient Asian secrets are and how they came to be adapted for today's beauty rituals. This chapter discusses how Koreans have traditionally defined beauty and how modern lifestyle ideas are changing and evolving—by impacting popular Korean beauty myths and practices today. Some practices are literally raising eyebrows and eyelids. Let's see why they have made Korea a haven for plastic surgery and the world's leader in this "beauty arena."

TRADITIONAL AND CURRENT IDEALS OF BEAUTY IN KOREA

We've shown in the previous chapter how research studies from Canadian and U.S. universities conclude that the beauty ideal for Asians from the Far East (and also one that's very universal around the world) is the age-old cultural preference for whiter, paler, and fairer skin. This is true for both men and women.

In Prof. Eric P. H. Li's cross-cultural analysis of advertisements for skin whitening products in India, Japan, Korea, and Hong Kong (along with his colleagues from these countries), women and men are more socially accepted based on lighter skin color.[31] Attractive looks matter, with a healthy glow for that deluxe touch.

In Korea, the standard is still for women to appear as "the fairer sex" in more ways than one. A flawless, porcelain-

---

[31] http://www.acrwebsite.org/volumes/v35/naacr_vol35_273.pdf

like facial complexion that's unblemished is *the* measure of beauty for which women strive. The traditional standard has always been milky skin that's polished and smooth as white jade—plus soft and dewy.

With such high aspirations for "perfect whiter beauty," it's not hard to see why the Korea Health Industry Development Institute reported that Korean women spent over $5.2 billion on beauty aids in 2009[32]—making South Korea the 12th largest cosmetics market in the world.

However, there is now literally a new wrinkle in Korean beauty standards—for aspiring beauty seekers to insert an extra eyelid fold through plastic surgery that's called blepharoplasty. Rhinoplasty, or nose jobs, too, are popular to straighten and raise noses with a pointy effect. With larger, rounder eyes and more aquiline bridges, many Koreans are looking more westernized.

Korean-American Julia Yoo noted in her blog that only about 25 percent of Koreans are born with the *ssang-ku-pool*, or crease above the eyelid.[33] When she was five, a family friend told Julia she had saved her parents lots of money. Translation? Her parents did not have to pay for a blepharoplasty.

According to Karyn Yun, director of L'Oreal Korea's Research and Development Center, "In Korea, more than 80 percent of people's interest in beauty has been on the face," with the remaining 20 percent on the body.[34] This contrasts sharply with Brazilian women, who apply cream all over their bodies, she notes.

Ms. Yun points out another cultural difference. Koreans prefer their skin tones a shade lighter than their original skin—in seeking "porcelain" shades. However, she finds

---

[32] http://joongangdaily.joins.com/article/view.asp?aid=2932534
[33]

http://web.mit.edu/cultureshock/fa2006/www/essays/koreanbeauty.html
[34] http://www.hancinema.net/korea-corners-the-market-on-beauty-6665.html

westerners like to match both face and body color—and usually go one tone darker to achieve this effect. Beauty is truly in the eye of the beholder.

When Julia Yoo visited Korea, she found cosmetic surgery to be a growing trend for men, too. Her then 29-year-old male cousin, who is slim and over six feet tall, got significantly more job offers than his best friend, who is shorter and heavier. Both men graduated with the same GPA from prestigious Seoul National University. For Korean men (as also true for their female counterparts), the two most popular procedures are eyelid and nose surgeries—in order to get ahead socially and professionally in landing jobs and promotions.[35]

Dr. Hyeonsook Lee, a dermatologist and cosmetic surgeon in Seoul's Gangnam district (where the majority of plastic surgery clinics are located in Korea), told me: "Generally, bald guys are under a lot of pressure in Korea. It's a throwback to traditional Korean standards of beauty because society loves black, rich hair. So there is a huge market for hair care products (medical and non-medical) for shampoo, conditioners and essences, herbal medicines, and including hair make-up."[36]

It's amazing this dermatologist mentions modern Korean cosmetic technology delivers instant "thick hair make-up" to augment the mane by spritzing it on—from spray cans. It's also a far cry from the 1800s, when she points out that the Korean beauty ideal of never cutting hair so it could grow "long, black, and rich" was celebrated every spring.

"Dano Day" fell on the fifth day of the fifth month of the year, when women would gather *chang-po* or calamus (*acorus calamus var. angustatus*), an aquatic herb growing in ponds and by shallow stream waters. *Chang-po* is an herbal

---

35

http://web.mit.edu/cultureshock/fa2006/www/essays/koreanbeauty.html
[36] Email received on 2/22/2011.

essence that's still a key ingredient in today's Korean shampoos and hair conditioners.

Dr. Lee lists hair transplants as one of top three beauty procedures performed in Korea. Not surprisingly, many Chinese men fly to Seoul to get hair transplants done, and very affordably, too. The other two popular beauty procedures are:

- Skin treatments—for acne, melasma, and skin rejuvenation. Dr. Lee's own specialty is treating these skin issues with laser and botox injections.

- Body sculpting—liposuction and fat transplantation or autologous fat injections, where excess fat from one area of the patient is transferred to another body area in the same patient.

In answer to my question on what women's beauty ideals are in Korea today, she notes: "In the early 1800s, a *mi-in-do*, or beautiful woman, would have a convex forehead, crescent-shaped eyebrows, single-fold eyelid, and small mouth. Today, one of Korea's most beautiful actresses—TV soap opera actress TaeHee Kim—has double-folded eyelids and eyebrows, a high and sharp nose, and a small oval-shaped face without the traditional square jaw line of Korean women."[37]

Dr. Lee further points out that the majority of Korean women (like women everywhere) are no less conscious of their bodies. "It is said that 80 percent of Korean women think they are overweight. As you know, Korean women are slim. And Korean celebrities are very thin. Nevertheless, they all want to be even slimmer and thinner. So liposuction is popular."[38]

---

[37] Email received on 2/23/2011.
[38] Email received on 2/22/2011.

ANCIENT KOREAN BEAUTY SECRETS

Longevity is an undeniable test of efficacy for any product. Let's look at some ancient Korean beauty secrets to see why, thousands of years later, they are still key beauty secrets. What is the folklore and cultural history behind the item? What are the benefits? Is there any science behind the benefits?

Ginseng

History. By all accounts, ginseng is thought to have originated in Korea and Manchuria (northern China). Revered as an overall tonic, the most important function of ginseng is to restore the body's health by rebalancing opposing, yet complementary, forces of yin and yang energies to promote the smooth flow of qi. Qi is the body's vital life force. When qi is unbalanced, immunity is lowered and sickness sets in. Ginseng was a precious and expensive elixir of life for royalty and the wealthy. Living up to its reputation, the ginseng plant can live for over a hundred years.

Benefits. Found only in Korean ginseng, it is rich in phytoestrogens called ginsenosides. Ginseng's health benefits[39] include:

- Increasing protein synthesis.
- Improving blood circulation and increasing blood supply.
- Improving brain function and memory with better blood flow.
- Reducing post-menopausal symptoms in women.
- Countering the effects of stress as an adaptogen.
- Anti-inflammatory effects.

---

[39] http://www.phytochemicals.info/plants/korean-ginseng.php

- Enhancing immune support for HIV-positive patients.
- Lowering blood glucose and the effects of insulin spikes for diabetic patients.
- Enhancing athletic performance as a natural anabolic steroid.
- Enhancing both male and female sexuality.

Scientific notes. The U.S. National Institutes of Health (NIH)'s National Center for Complementary and Alternative Medicine Web site has an informative fact sheet.[40] MedlinePlus, a service of the NIH's U.S. National Library of Science, also lists pros and cons on its Web site.[41] Western science is still researching the effects of ginseng.

Meantime, Jill Blakeway, founder of New York City's YinOva Center, explains that ginseng's medicinal properties reflect the Korean medical concept of *Sang Seng*. When the body's opposing energies of yin and yang are harmonized by a tonic such as ginseng and other complementary herbs, the person's well-being is reflected in their inner health and radiant outer beauty.[42]

Black Beans

Who knew the humble black bean packs such potent punches for health and beauty? In Korea, black beans have had a long history of maintaining the beauty standard for "black, rich hair." The Japanese also love black beans for health, beauty and vitality.

History. A dietary protein staple in many Asian, African, and South American countries, black beans offer amazing health benefits. When the body is well-nourished with good food, lustrous skin and thick shiny hair mirror the person's

---

[40] http://nccam.nih.gov/health/asianginseng/ataglance.htm
[41] http://www.nlm.nih.gov/medlineplus/druginfo/natural/1000.html
[42] http://www.yinovacenter.com/blog/archives/5677/

inner well-being and an honest measure of good health and true beauty radiate from within.

Benefits. Black beans are superfoods! Called the "poor person's meat," black beans are nutritiously dense with goodness, such as:

- Renowned as free radical scavengers, black beans reduce oxidative effects, which wreak havoc on body and skin cells—making them anti-aging and anti-carcinogenic.
- Rich in protein, a dish of black beans combined with whole brown rice is comparable to meat and dairy foods—and without saturated fats and extra calories.
- Fiber-rich, black beans balance blood sugar and remove cholesterol.
- Heart-friendly in lowering the risks of heart attacks.

Scientific notes. According to researchers at Michigan State University, black beans are rich in antioxidants called anthocyanins. These findings were published in the *Journal of Agriculture and Food Chemistry* (November, 2003).[43] Similar findings of black beans having the highest sources of anthocyanins are supported by research at the University of Guelph, Ontario, Canada.[44] (Anthocyanins are also found in darker-colored fruit, such as blueberries and grapes.)

FIR (Far Infrared Rays)

Koreans have long understood how far infrared rays (FIR) rejuvenate body cells on deeper levels for longer-lasting effects. While the human body does emit FIR, stress, illness, and other factors can bring on imbalances. That's where saunas emitting FIR externally complements and helps

---

[43] http://happynutritionist.com/blackbeans.html
[44] http://www.todaysseniorsnetwork.com/healthy_beans.htm

promote healing on the body's deeper levels—and are common in Korean-style spas.[45]

Sauna chambers are built with natural clay, salt, and mineral stones, such as jade. My friend, June Kwon, has kindly described four Korean healing chambers:

1. Salt brick. Salt can become a powerful remedy, if used properly. Heart muscles continuously circulate blood while consuming this mineral. A shortage leads to excreting less urine, resulting in less toxins excreted—which causes a toxic buildup in the body. Made from 350-million-year-old salt rocks, this room rejuvenates skin. (115~120 degrees Fahrenheit)

2. Red clay. Unique to ancient Korean culture, this room combines the benefits of infrared rays and the absorptive nature of yellow soil to extract toxins from within the body. (120~125 degrees Fahrenheit)

3. Jade. Jade contains magnesium, iron, and calcium essential for the body. Jade radiates infrared rays that help discharge internal toxins, neutralize blood to become more alkaline, and re-activates bodily rhythms. Jade also increases brain activity, enhances the nervous system, and prevents osteoporosis.

4. Ice. Chilled to just above freezing, a brisk cold treatment stimulates blood flow and tightens the skin. (35 degrees Fahrenheit)

For example, Olympus Spas has two locations: south of Seattle (which started in 1997) and north in Lynnwood (opened in 2005). Both introduced FIR's deeper dermal healing concepts to their women-only Korean-style bathhouses.

The *Seattle Times*' featured Olympus Spa in its Sunday weekly magazine, *Pacific Northwest* (9/21/2003).[46] In its article

---

[45] http://www.olympusspa.net/Tacoma/news-detail.aspx?newsid=96

written by the newspaper's Korean-American reporter Paula Bock, she explains it's a cultural tradition dating back over 2,000 years where: "Women—all kinds of women—soak, scrub, steam, and relax, a tradition spanning centuries and the globe, evolved from times when few families had their own private bath."

Lilo, a German quoted in this article, says, "The steam rooms and hot rooms are really about detoxification. When you release toxins, not just on a physical level, but also on a mental-emotional level, you get in a space of relaxation and you forget about your daily worries. I feel like a new person when I leave there."

The hot or heat rooms Lilo mentions are warmed up by FIR or far infrared rays. Unlike solar rays, which burn skin easily, FIR enhances blood circulation, expels toxins, and promotes cellular production in bones and muscles, too.

Olympus Spa manager Sun Lee is emphatic about FIR's myriad health and beauty benefits for women. For example, he cites the jade room as promoting cellular healing while purifying the entire body to maintain total body health and wellness. Moreover, Sun Lee explains FIR breaks down fat cells, stabilizes bodily functions, normalizes blood pressure, and activates collagen production—all the right reasons for women who *want* health and beauty goals to bless their lives.

It's interesting to me how Korean-style saunas and spas such as Olympus are now setting the standard for healing and maintaining natural wellness in this country. I previously mentioned a *Los Angeles Times*[47] article (12/20/2010) discussing natural Korean healing using herbal remedies for the vaginal path. This article reports that Deangki Spa in LA's Koreatown charges "$20 a squat," while Juvenex Spa[48] in

---

[46] http://seattletimes.nwsource.com/pacificnw/2003/0921/cover.html

[47] http://articles.latimes.com/2010/dec/20/health/la-he-v-steam-20101220

[48] http://www.juvenexspa.com/html/services_menu/specialtytreatments.html#GYNO SPA CURE

Manhattan's Koreatown offers a 30-minute "Gyno-Spa Cure" for $75.

Called *chai-york* in Korean, it's also offered in Santa Monica, California, at Tikkun Spa, owned by Niki Han Schwarz and her orthopedic surgeon husband, Charles. Their "V-Steam" ($50 for 30 minutes) is an ancient ritual stimulating hormones to do their job, specifically in maintaining uterine health, menstrual cycles, correcting digestive disorders, and soothing the nervous system.[49] The two primary herbs are mugwort and wormwood. Being anti-bacterial and anti-fungal, these two herbs promote internal health, plus "keep your skin looking young," this Web site offers.

Niki Han Schwarz found that after five V-steams, she had fewer body aches—plus more energy. And she was finally able to conceive at age 45, after having tried unsuccessfully for three years to get pregnant!

This *LA Times* article quoted Dr. Suzanne Gilberg-Lenz of Women's Care at the Beverly Hills' Medical Group as calling *chai-york* "not insane" because steaming the pelvic area with medicinal herbs: 1) introduces heat; 2) boosts blood circulation; and 3) enhances "immune factors" into the lower part of the body.

It's worth reiterating how beauty and health standards change as they evolve to meet current needs. The bottom line? Men and women *always* want to look their healthiest best.

When you attain confidence from looking healthy and nicely put together, it shows—and gets you ahead professionally, socially, and emotionally.

---

[49] http://www.tikkunspa.com/images/pdfs/Tikkun_SpaMenu.pdf

KOREAN BEAUTY TREATMENTS TODAY THRIVE ON TRADITIONAL HEALING CONCEPTS

As a Korean-born physician and Cornell University-trained dermatologist, I'm especially interested in why and how age-old beauty and health philosophies from this culture are so enduring—and endearing—for women and men today. I've explained why New York City's top beauty emporium Bergdorf Goodman proudly introduced the first-ever totally herbal-based cosmetics in 2010—the Sulwhasoo Concentrated Ginseng Cream, costing $220 an ounce.[50]

Indeed, when we peel back the outer layers of cosmetic and plastic appearances, I'm thrilled to find the science behind Korean cosmetics validated.

For instance, New York City's top beauty emporium Berdorf Goodman cites Korea's *Donguibogam* as a solid foundation for the development of health and beauty principles in Korea.[51] In essence, quality Korean cosmetics are based on traditional herbal healing and medicinal practices. *Bogam*, as this 25-volume encyclopedia of medical healing is commonly called, is a treasure trove of ancient Korean beauty secrets.

Therefore, even as Koreans embrace modern-day plastic surgery for all the allure and professional enhancements cosmetic corrections can gift them, I'm delighted to find ancient, natural herbal and medicinal remedies for beauty treatments to be very much alive now—in nurturing easterners and westerners.

The integrity and enriching legacy of ancient Korean medical sciences and herbal healing now utilized by modern scientists integrating centuries-old "secrets" in formulating

---

[50] Price listed in February 2011;
http://blog.bergdorfgoodman.com/womens-style/sulwhasoo
[51] http://portal.unesco.org/ci/en/files/27075/12133693253Korea_Dong uibogam.pdf/Korea%2BDonguibogam.pdf

beauty innovations for today's demanding consumers is priceless.

I also recognize the inter-connectedness of Korean, Japanese, and Chinese healing concepts. The vaginal steam using mugwort and woodworm herbs offered in Korean-style spas today first came to light in the Chinese *Compendium of Materia Medica,* compiled by Li Shizhen during the Ming Dynasty (1368-1644). As Qing Yan, M.D., Ph.D., notes in his book, *Herbs for Beauty: Imperial and Secret Herbal Formulas from Ancient China* (2005)[52], the Chinese followed the tradition of bathing with these herbs on the fifth day of the fifth month—to "expel wind, eliminate sputum, and alleviate itching and pain." It's similar to ancient Koreans celebrating "Dano Day" on this same day when the herbal remedy *chang-po* was gathered from shallow stream waters for herbal hair essences.

THREE KOREAN ANCIENT BEAUTY SECRETS

- Herbal Secrets. Korean scientists are savvy in incorporating medicinal herbal practices based on ancient wisdom for contemporary cosmetics. For instance, Korea's reputation in growing superior ginseng enables it to produce naturally effective herbal healing creams—without chemical enhancements—to the delight of anti-aging fans.

- Dermal Heating Secrets. FIR (for infrared rays) is a wonderful example of a centuries-old Korean innovation accessing deep dermal heat for healing body and skin issues that is still very effective for all the health and healing issues listed above.

- Holistic Applications. Korean, Japanese, and Chinese beauty and health secrets are inter-related. Proven

---

[52] Page 74.

through thousands of years of efficacious use, they are now validated by modern science applications.

> *"My mother installed in us that nourishing the inner beauty is just as important as taking care of the outer beauty. She made us eat healthy foods like walnuts, as well as protect our skin with plenty of sun protection. As she said, beauty comes from the inside and out."*
>
> — Min Kim-Lee, Korean Actress, Los Angeles, CA

CHAPTER THREE

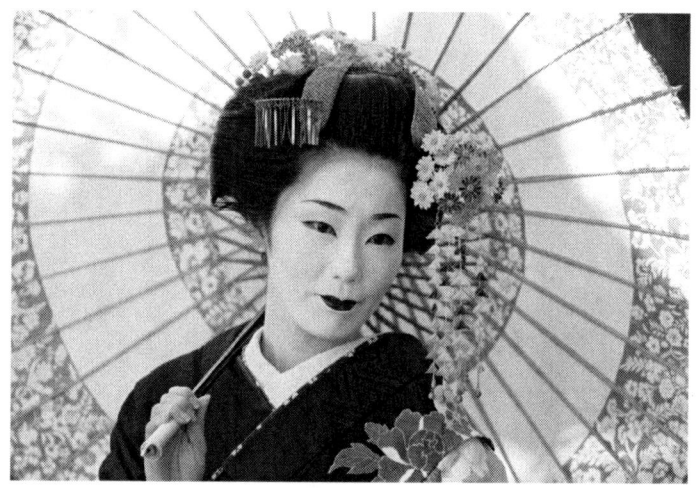

3

How is Beauty Defined in Japan?

Japan has a long history of appreciating beauty—from the geisha culture to traditional crafts. Their spa culture is thousands of years old, and traditional ingredients such as volcanic mud, wakame seaweed, rice bran, and even nightingale droppings have been shown to have skin benefits (the bird droppings, long used by geisha and kabuki actors, contain the enzyme guanine, which brightens the skin).

Renowned for their high-tech performance, Japanese brands nevertheless offer a holistic approach, using elements of traditional Eastern medicine and aromachology. Last year, Uemura launched a skincare range, Phyto-Black Lift, using ingredients such as hyaluronic acid and glycoaminoglycan, to help firm and moisturise the skin. But it's the quirkier ingredients, fermented black tea and black sugar, that tell the magical story. The packaging says: "In the fifth century, the Japanese emperor was cured from sickness and lived long thanks to the mystic beverage, black tea ferment, made with black tea and sugar.

Since those days, Japanese people believe that black ingredients such as black tea and black sugar is the key to stay young and healthy."
　　　　—Kristy Munro[53], *Brisbane Times* (10/22/2008),
　　　　　　　　　　　　　　　　　　　　Australia

---

[53] http://www.brisbanetimes.com.au/news/beauty/japan-embraces-its-inner-geisha/2008/10/22/1224351313363.html

A MERICAN ANTHROPOLOGIST LIZA DALBY'S firsthand and first-rate account of her yearlong stint as Geisha Ichigiku in the "flower and willow world" of Kyoto's Pontochô geisha community is a wondrous book. Geisha[54] reveals a closeted and credentialed club of talented entertainers who remain unmarried—as lifelong women companions to Japan's male elites. Geishas dance, sing, play musical instruments, write poetry and literary prose, plus perform the traditional Japanese tea ceremony for guests.

The geisha profession began in the 1800s. Soon, geishas became style-setters and fashion arbiters to Japanese women. However, living the geisha lifestyle of disciplined glamour came at a price—geishas cannot marry. Instead, they take lovers or bear the children of their patrons, or *danna*. "The ideal of artistic achievement and feminine allure that they represent is deeply rooted in Japan," Liza observes.[55] Liza's groundbreaking book was published in 1983. Geisha culture today is still flourishing with its allure of artistic graces and stylish beauty.

When I asked Liza about Japanese beauty ideals, she told me, "As you know, geishas hate to get sun-tanned. White skin is, of course, a traditional attribute of feminine beauty in Japan. Even when they are not wearing the white face paint (*o-shiroi*) that goes on with the wig and formal costume, they prefer naturally pale skin."[56] This was also mentioned earlier in Prof. Paul Li, et. al.'s research that Japanese men prefer their women *mochi-hada*—or skin like pounded rice—and the cultural preference for smooth, silky, supple, and whitened female skin.[57]

Incredibly, Japan's beauty trends are arcing back to history with "an interest in traditional cosmetics," Liza said. "In the 1970s, foreign brands were big. But now, Japanese

---

[54] http://lizadalby.com/LD/Geisha_info.html
[55] Email from Liza Dalby, 2/20/2011.
[56] Ibid.
[57] http://www.acrwebsite.org/volumes/v35/naacr_vol35_273.pdf

brands have at least as much cachet. Shiseido and Kanebo offer various skin whiteners that geisha, as well as ordinary Japanese women, use."

A similar analysis of Japanese beauty ideals returning to tried and true ancient secrets is reported in an article by Stephanie Rafanelli in London's newspaper *Daily Mail*, "Turning Japanese: beauty that's taking over." (June 25, 2007)[58].

"Japan's cultural obsession with flawless skin, youth and purification, has made beauty big business with more people working in the industry than wedding and funeral services, auto-repair and the software industries combined. And we in the West are only just beginning to catch up as we become more youth orientated and aware of the benefits of natural products," Stephanie writes.

What gives? She quotes Krista Madden, editor of www.beautyandthedirt.co.ok: "We've all heard about potentially harmful chemical anti-aging agents that can be absorbed through the skin. Now, the tide has turned to natural, earthy treatments that have been tried and tested by women over centuries. (Besides) Japanese beauty products focus on anti-aging and sun damage. The Japanese beauty industry has always concentrated on lightening the skin, because pure, white, unblemished skin is prized above all things."

According to Stefanie, the benchmark of Japanese beauty is: "A look of sexual innocence with pale, unblemished skin and shiny, silky hair." Simply natural.

Japanese women find their own nature-based beauty products worthy of spending over $26 billion annually, reports the *Wall Street Journal* (12/22/2010),[59] which makes

---

[58] http://www.dailymail.co.uk/femail/article-464194/Turning-Japanese-beauty-thats-taking-over.html
[59] http://online.wsj.com/article/SB10001424052748703581204576033401654446640.html?KEYWORDS=japanese+beauty+products

the Japanese cosmetics market the second largest in the world.

Japanese beauty websites are gold mines of authentic information, too. Ancient Japanese beauty products are explained with delightful historical anecdotes at:

- www.naturaljapanesebeauty.com, which sells a range of nature-based skin care made from seaweed, nightingale droppings, to green tea;

- www.camelliaoil.com has charming historical beauty tips for *camellia japonica*; plus nuggets, such as using boxwood combs to avoid split ends for hair—apparently, no one reported this problem during the Edo Dynasty (17th-19th centuries), and beautiful long hair was very much *en vogue* then.

Let us see how and why these ancient Japanese secrets endure—as modern science races in the opposite direction with laboratory-based, nano-tech experiments for beauty products. The Japanese are renowned for leading-edge innovations based on thoughtful applications that meet real needs.

FROM MOTHER NATURE'S BEAUTY PANTRY

Tsubaki or Camellia Oil

History. Since the Heian period (8th-12th centuries), *tsubaki* oil has moistened glowing skin and hair by bestowing a lustrous sheen on a person's crowning glory. Lightly fragrant, camellia oil is higher in oleic acids than olive oil—making it a super heart-healthy and light cooking oil that complements digestion, too. We are what we eat; with internal and external health bolstered by this one remarkable oil, lucky consumers of *tsubaki* have much for which to thank Mother Nature.

Benefits. We briefly discussed camellia oil's many plusses in Chapter One, including: a) moisturizes oily skin without clogging pores, b) naturally fades stretch marks and acne scars, c) heals burns, d) softens cuticles and e) promotes glossy hair growth without making it greasy.[60]

Nuka or Rice Bran

History. Japanese women have been reaping the benefits of bathing with water used for washing rice for centuries—with stunning results in showcasing smooth, supple, blemish-free, and porcelain-like whitened skin.

Benefits. Paul Pitchford, author of *Healing with Whole Foods*, defines unrefined brown rice bran as "one of the most nutrient dense substances ever studied."[61]

Scientific notes. Paul Pitchfird reports rice bran has over 70 antioxidants that protect against cellular damage and, therefore, preserve skin's youthfulness. *Nuka* has alpha-lipoic acid (ALA), a polyphenol antioxidant that promotes liver restoration, slows the aging process, and converts glucose to energy—in addition to myriad properties, such as wound healing and anti-aging.

Bamboo Sap

History. Long revered as "divine water" by the ancients, bamboo sap is a hydrating superhero fluid that reenergizes skin vitality.

Benefits. Bamboo sap is enriched with essential minerals such as potassium, magnesium, and iron to stimulate skin elasticity; has nine essential amino acids needed to build protein blocks and strengthen skin; and saccharides to

---

[60] http://www.iheartdaily.com/2009/11/japanese-beauty-secret-camellia-oil.html
[61] Page 13. Paul Pitchford's list of rice bran benefits.

energize skin cells. Bamboo sap is a true beauty aid from nature's own pharmacy.

Scientific notes. Even French cosmetics company Roger & Gallet has a large selection of products incorporating the benefits of bamboo sap for its powerful re-mineralizing properties and sugars—notably, a vegetal base treatment restoring elasticity and suppleness to the skin.[62]

FROM MOTHER NATURE'S FOOD PANTRY

Green Tea

History. Although tea (*camellia sinensis*) was serendipitously discovered by Chinese Emperor Shen Nong 5,000 years ago, unfermented green tea is now a Japanese superhero. Anti-aging and great for facial packs, green tea paste gently heals skin lesions, as well.

Benefits. Paul Pitchford describes some highlights of green tea in: a) opening up acupuncture meridians, b) improving digestion, c) being good for chronic inflammation, d) invigorating the constitution, and e) serving as an astringent to dry skin conditions like herpes and poison oak/ivy outbreaks.[63]

A Japanese friend, Naoko Tani-Fukuchi tells me, "Japanese green tea peeling gel keeps my skin in good condition. I use absolutely no makeup."

Scientific notes. The University of Maryland Medical Center has an informative Web site describing the healing benefits of polyphenols in green tea enjoyed by millions around the world. Polyphenols neutralize free radicals which wreak havoc on body cells.[64]

---

[62] http://www.shoplondons.com/bamboo.html
[63] Page 209. *Healing with Whole Foods*.
[64] http://www.umm.edu/altmed/articles/green-tea-000255.htm

Adzuki or **Red Beans**

History. A protein staple common in Japanese and Chinese cooking for the past few hundred years (after its introduction from South America), ground *adzuki* bean is a great skin exfoliant, too.

Benefits. Rich in saponins or natural plant detergents that do *not* strip away essential oils while exfoliating skin, red beans are also moisturizing. It's easy to make your own cleanser with organic red beans by cleaning them well and grinding them finely in a blender or grinder. Mix into a paste with water to apply and rinse off, or leave on for 10 to 15 minutes for a cooling facial.

Scientific notes. Adzuki or red beans are protein-rich, full of protease inhibitors which assist in fighting pathogens, and a great fiber food.[65]

Umeboshi or **Pickled Plums**

History. Organic umeboshi has long been a Japanese alkalizing and medicinal cure-all for every conceivable situation and malaise.[66] My friend Erika Erickson, who is Japanese, advises, "An umeboshi a day keeps the doctor away."

Benefits. From promoting food freshness in lunch boxes to good digestion, pickled plums build up body fluids, which in turn moisturize body and skin cells and boost liver function. However, Paul Pitchford warns that too much of a good thing can backfire—in this case, since umeboshi is rich in oxalic acid, they can deplete the body's calcium.[67]

Scientific notes. Powerfully acidic, umeboshi plays a powerfully paradoxical role in alkalinizing foods—in

---

[65] http://fitho.in/guide/beans/adzuki-beans/
[66] http://www.mitoku.com/products/umeboshi/healthbenefits.html
[67] Page 623. *Healing with Whole Foods.*

stimulating digestion, eliminating toxins, and providing the body with more energy.[68]

Seaweed

History. A country of islands, Japan is naturally rich in marine algae. Men and women have been eating copious amounts of this healing and longevity secret for centuries. Nori, hijiki, and wakame are among the more common seaweeds.

Benefits. Paul Pitchford lists more plusses for seaweed, in: a) detoxifying, b) moistening dryness and building up yin body fluids, c) softening hardened areas in the body, d) removing radiation in the body, e) alkalizing the blood, f) activating liver qi, g) lowering cholesterol, and h) possessing soothing, mucilaginous gels, such as algin, carrageenan, and agar, which rejuvenate the lungs and gastro-intestinal tract.[69]

Scientific notes. Minerals in seaweed promote shiny, strong hair. Best of all, seaweed is rich in hyaluronic acid that keeps skin moisturized—and is a great anti-aging agent in reducing dry skin and wrinkles, while promoting soft, supple skin.[70] Korea is also big on consuming seaweeds for health reasons and culinary enjoyment.

Miso

History. Naturally fermented soybeans pack powerful punches of probiotic enzymes. Naturally aged in huge wooden vats for a few months up to a few years, boiling destroys the enzymes. Miso is only stirred in after the ingredients have cooked, while the soup is still hot, but not boiling. Miso is also protein-rich with nutrients and minerals.

---

[68] http://www.mitoku.com/products/umeboshi/healthbenefits.html
[69] Page 581; ibid.
[70] http://seaweedskin.com/

Soy Beans

History. Soy is an ancient Far Eastern food secret promoting good health and smooth skin—and is a very affordable protein (38 percent).

Benefits. Paul Pitchford lists their many benefits: a) have more protein than milk, without the saturated fat or cholesterol, b) moistens dryness, c) supplements the kidneys, d) improves circulation, e) highly alkalizing, f) detoxifying, g) restores pancreatic functions for diabetics, h) boosts milk production for nursing mothers, and finally, i) a remedy for skin eruptions.[71]

Mushrooms

History. In Far Eastern medicine, mushrooms are renowned as "the medicine of kings." Andrew Weil, M.D., the world's leading integrative health expert incorporating allopathic and naturopathic healing modalities, has developed a beauty care line using reishi mushrooms (an ancient Asian staple) for Origins, one of America's earliest cosmetics companies selling nature-based products.

Benefits. Origins' Plantidote™ item uses "mushroom magic," such as reishi and cordyceps, to provide relief for red and sensitive skin. It "is designed to tame inflammation, which, according to Weil, can cause puffiness, wrinkles and fine lines, as well as dry, red skin," writes Laurel Vukovic for CBS' moneywatch.com.[72]

Scientific notes. Two other edible fungus delicacies promoting beauty from inside out are maitake and shiitake; being tasty only enhances their health, beauty, and culinary allure.[73]

---

[71] Page 510; ibid.
[72] http://findarticles.com/p/articles/mi_m0FKA/is_2_69/ai_n27125054/
[73] http://www.naturalnews.com/021498.html

From Mother Nature's Unlimited Cosmic Stores of Energy

An endearing aspect of ancient societies is recognizing nature's impact on daily living. Even with her 21st century technological prowess, Japan is ever cognizant of subtle energy shifts exerted by the environment and seasons on their culture.

It is not surprising that in a land bereft of minerals and other natural resources, people have delved deeper to resourcefully harness nature's intangible gifts—that is, prevailing upon subtle energy shifts to revitalize body and spirit, and sharing the precious wealth of living in peace and prosperity with one another.

Shun ("shoon") Food

<u>History.</u> In Japan, *food is medicine.* In Japanese gastronomy, the chef's daily menu (*kaiseki*) offers seasonal foods that are also locally sourced. Why? Because food that has to travel loses valuable nutrients while in transit. More importantly, over the centuries, the Japanese have astutely noticed subtle energy fluctuations in nature every 10 days.

<u>Benefits.</u> Therefore, eating fresh, healthy foods alive with nature's seasonal energies is half the battle won in helping the body stay healthy.

<u>Scientific notes.</u> The Japanese honor Shun foods because they subtly enhance health and culinary enjoyment by capturing nature's freshest seasonal foods.[74]

Tea Ceremony

<u>History.</u> The art of Chado or Way of Tea was introduced from China over a thousand years ago to Buddhist temples in Japan.

---

[74] http://www.japanesefoodculture.org/food/culture.html

Benefits. This gracious aesthetic lifestyle ceremony honors friends by sharing green tea and sweet cakes in meditative practice that went beyond temple walls. The uninitiated may find it challenging to sit cross-legged for an extended period. However, the serenity of a living meditation art form can be life-altering, as Chado enthusiasts and converts show. A heartfelt experience all its own, "*Chanoyu* should be made with the heart, not with the hand. Make it without making it, in the stillness of your mind," advises Hamamoto Shoshun, Urasenke Tradition Chado senior instructor.

Scientific notes. Heartfelt love and sincere friendship *are* silent and eloquent expressions with Chado—while rebalancing body and spirit harmoniously for host and guests in soulful meditation. "Serious practitioners can ... transform tension-producing details of everyday life into moments of beauty, meaningfulness, and tranquility."[75]

Shiatsu

Japanese bodywork is similar to Chinese acupressure. Both aim to unclog energy flows in meridians for qi to flow and rebalance the body's internal harmony. Shiatsu practitioners use fingers and the pressure from their palms to help along energy flow.

Reiki

History. "Rei" means God's Higher Power in Japanese, while "ki" means life force, as in qi. Discovered by Dr. Mikao Usui in March 1922, reiki works through energy channels similar to the "laying of hands" in effecting healing where needed on the body.[76]

Benefits. Non-invasive, reiki is a popular technique that transfers healing energy to patients.

---

[75] http://www.ncbi.nlm.nih.gov/pubmed/8550688
[76] http://www.reiki.org/faq/HistoryOfReiki.html#usui

<u>Scientific notes.</u> The National Center for Complementary and Alternative Medicine (an arm of the U.S. National Institutes of Health) categorizes reiki as a form of energy medicine, along with qi gong, therapeutic touch, and electro-magnetic therapy.[77]

Yukkuri tanoshiko

Slow down, enjoy it. That's right. Take time to enjoy "The Moment." While a person outside of Japanese culture might see it as a waste of time to enjoy "empty moments," traditionally, Japanese people love to experience the exact opposite—enjoying moments of quiet serendipity and being resuscitated by them emotionally and mentally. Making time for down time to rebalance our energies is a more productive use of time, when wisely spent.

WHAT'S INSPIRING ABOUT JAPANESE BEAUTY SECRETS?

- Eating wisely enhances beauty and health. Plus, it *is* a conscious choice in that everyone has total control over what they select as the most nourishing for them—not only food-wise, but emotionally, mentally, physically, and spiritually.

- The courage to recognize the wisdom of ancient beauty secrets, regardless of what modern science may unfold with more expensive, nano-based cosmetics.

- Integrating meditative practices into harried lifestyles to rebalance body-mind-spirit for total well-being and in looking naturally beautiful—with radiant beauty shining forth that's reflected in soft, dewy skin.

---

[77] http://en.wikipedia.org/wiki/Energy_medicine

The most important internal act we can do to enhance our beauty is practice compassion—first for ourselves, then to others. To reach out to those who might seem the least likely to be messengers/teachers; because their diversity of experience, background and culture may bring about the most enlightening truths about our own self and our own need to grow.

It has been important for me to learn that I must constantly work to re-invent or re-create myself, and be open to the stories of all people. It is in the act of opening oneself that beauty is truly revealed to us, and from us.

—Janice Mirikitani, Poet Laureate of San Francisco

CHAPTER FOUR

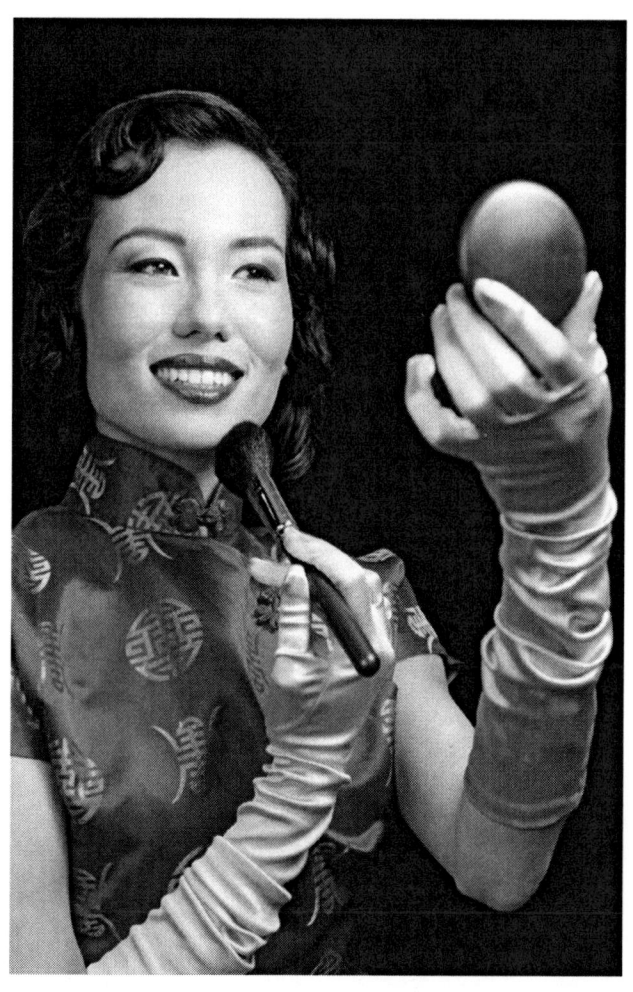

4

How is Beauty Defined in China?

The effects of FRA (Facial Revitalization Acupuncture) vary according to the prior condition and lifestyle of the patient, the techniques employed by the practitioner, as well as the experience and skill level of the practitioner. Although one cannot promise or guarantee results or advertise as such, FRA may erase as many as five to fifteen years from the face, with some results apparent as early as the first treatment. The effects of acupuncture being cumulative, the results continue to progress throughout the course of treatment.

Though not a cure for wrinkles, fine lines may be eliminated while deeper wrinkles tend to diminish considerably. Other likely results include eyebags being reduced or eliminated, puffiness of the face reduced or banished, facial coloring equalized (whether too red or too pale), drooping eyelids lifted, and double chins minimized and in some cases eliminated. Drooping eyelids and eyebrows, jowls and 'turkey necks' can be observed as having lifted and toned. With the profound increase of local circulation of qi *and blood to the face and stimulation of the movement of lymph, skin texture and coloring improves visibly, the moisture content of the skin improves, muscle tone improves, and pore size is regulated. Techniques can also be employed to eliminate broken capillaries. Rosacea may also respond to FRA treatment in certain cases that I have seen. Visible stress and habitual expressions from the face melt away. By balancing* qi, *blood, fluids, and* yin *and* yang, *the body is put into balance and optimum tone so that the ageing process and its causes are slowed down, halted or even reversed.*

As with regular acupuncture, the results are manifold and include the improvement of circulation, digestion and hormonal balance, and empirically have been found to benefit the hair and the sense organs, thyroid and brain.

—Virginia Doran, European Journal of Oriental Medicine[78]

I N ANCIENT CHINA, THE land of bound feet and breasts, beauty ideals were never sensual or overtly sexy. Instead, beauty standards were artistic, rather than showing off a woman's face. Just as young men aspired to imperial offices by taking rigorous annual examinations, young women who aspired to become royal concubines had to be tested on math, literature, and the arts—in order to win the emperor's favors.

For those not so fortunate in winning imperial favors, Chinese women were extolled to possess "Ten Criteria for Beauty in Ancient China." According to Huo Jianying, they were[79]:

1. Black lustrous hair and temples "as thin as cicada wings."
2. Loosely coiled hair on top of the head for an illusion of added height.
3. Finely shaped eyebrows.
4. Large, bright expressive eyes.
5. Red lips and white teeth for health and beauty.
6. Graceful, slim, and soft fingers with fair and fleshy arms.
7. Slender waist and fair skin, with a willowy illusion.
8. Tiny feet and a light, elegant gait.
9. Dressing appropriately.
10. A clean, fragrant body.

---

[78] http://www.ejom.co.uk/vol-5-no-5/featured-articles/
[79] http://www.chinatoday.com.cn/English/p58.htm

Front and center, a woman's crowning glory consisted of a shiny mane and attractive facial features; followed by a cultural preference for a slim, willowy figure; down to tiny feet and an elegant gait. A woman's hands were considered her "second face." To round off her beauteous presentation, a Chinese woman was expected to dress appropriately and to be cleanly scented.

It appears history (or her-story) repeats itself as these criteria continue to resonate as strongly today. Cosmeticsdesigns.com reported cosmetics sales in China reached $10.8 billion in 2009. RNCOS estimates China's skin and hair care industry to exceed $25 billion in 2012.[80] Many beauty formulations continue to depend on centuries-old "secret" beauty ingredients. What were they?

As I've mentioned in the Introduction, ancient Asian beauty secrets relied on three main categories to heal and beautify the body by:

- Rebalancing the body's energies with qi energy work, such as acupuncture and acupressure, so qi flows naturally for optimal health.
- Nourishing the body with good food for good health so natural beauty is a shining reflection of the body's internal health.
- Relying on animal- and nature-based herbs and tonics to rejuvenate body and skin.

The plant and animal kingdoms, in tune with naturally adapting to Mother Nature's spontaneous and fluctuating seasons, plus environmental changes, became nature's healing apothecary in restoring vitality and radiant beauty for bodies besieged by climatic elements.

This classical recipe for Far Eastern Asian health secrets began over 5,000 years ago in China—then was adapted in

---

[80] http://www.cosmeticsdesign.com/Business-Financial/China-cosmetic-sales-growth-powers-ahead-but-rate-slows

Korea and Japan. Renowned today as a powerful healing force, Traditional Chinese Medicine, or TCM, is embraced by Western medical practitioners, as well. Let's examine some of these amazing ancient Chinese healing remedies that are also vital to Asian beauty secrets.

THE ROLE OF TCM FOR SKIN BEAUTY

First, let us briefly discuss Traditional Chinese Medicine. The fundamental tenet of TCM celebrates wellness when the body is in total harmony—in optimally harnessing opposing, yet complementary, forces of yin and yang. As I've also mentioned, it's a state of *wu-wei* when a healthy body goes with the flow of external forces, such as adapting to nature's seasons and environmental changes. Therefore, when the body is healthy, imbalances are naturally and quickly restored to maintain homeostasis or a state of dynamic equilibrium.

However, imbalances can also occur for prolonged onslaughts by pathogens (such as bacteria, viruses, fungus, chemical pesticides, genetically modified foods, and nuclear radiation) in assaulting the complementary forces of yin-yang. When imbalances are not restored, the body's harmonious integrity or cycle of good health is broken. That's when we feel "dis-ease" with the body's immune system compromised—in making it more susceptible to pathogenic invasions, such as colds and coughs, not to mention more serious diseases over time, given the long-term accumulations of pathogens.

A TCM physician diagnoses the root cause(s) after identifying which ones to treat—and employs a very different clinical approach from western medicine, which treats symptoms. The primary goal in TCM is to customize treatment, as each patient responds differently to pathogens and prescriptions.

How are TCM treatments customized? An ancient Chinese medicine saying goes: *Same disease; different treatment. Same treatment; different disease.*

Meaning, there are myriad ways to root out pathogens for restoring good health.

For various patients manifesting one same skin problem, such as acne, there would *not* be a one-size-fits-all tube of ointment to apply. Instead, various herbal concoctions would be devised according to a patient's specific needs.

Along with herbal medicines, acupuncture would also be administered to unclog qi, the primal life force in all living things. Flowing qi in turn reactivates healing energy to course through the body again, functionally, as it's intended to—for example, unclogging blood circulation, which helps produce new elastin and collagen production for new, smooth skin. Once internal harmony is restored in the body, it's reflected in overall good outer health and clear, glowing skin.

An added advantage is that Chinese herbal remedies do not typically incur side effects. However, as acupuncturist and Chinese herbalist Jill Blakeway points out, although tonifying herbs like ginseng do strengthen immunity, they can also strengthen pathogens once they've overtaken the body's resistance. She advises taking a break from herbs and restarting after two symptom-free days.[81] She also advises consulting with a TCM practitioner with more than ten years' experience.

At Jill's YinOva Center clinic in New York City, renowned for her expertise in using TCM to help women conceive, she also treats skin problems. In Chapter One, I noted her skin strategy in cleansing the liver, as this is the body's first line of defense in detoxifying impurities from the blood. Clean blood that circulates robustly is vital for body cells to keep on regenerating.

---

[81] http://yinovacenter.com/wp-content/uploads/Jill-NAT-HEALTH-NOVEMBER-20093.pdf

Jill notes that as women age, the body's yin energy diminishes, which results in skin becoming drier, less elastic, and more inflamed. She recommends soothing red and irritated skin with a high-quality ginseng cream.

Jill points out, too, that ginseng is a great adaptogen herb in helping women adapt to stress, fatigue, and pollution; it can be taken orally by cooking it in soups and stews, or simply boiling ginseng root in filtered water for a clear tea to sip.[82]

Additionally, another pathogen recognized by TCM to impact illness is stress on the body—emotional and continuously strenuous physical labor. But this condition is reversible by making down time to rest, exercise with tai chi or qi gong, or with silent meditation.

ANCIENT CHINESE BEAUTY SECRETS

Let's now see how Chinese beauty secrets came about with energy work, which have been developing TCM healing modalities for over 5,000 years.

Acupuncture

History. With over 5,000 years of history behind it, acupuncture has developed many applications. Fine, sterile hair-thin needles are inserted to correct the flow of qi at various pressure points to rebalance internal harmony to facilitate the body's recovery.

Benefits. A popular acupuncture application is facial rejuvenation. The Chinese discovered that meridian points begin in the face and course on throughout the body. Apparently:

---

[82] http://www.style.com/beauty/beautycounter/2010/11/a-healer-walks-among-us/#more-5774

- eyelids and eyebrows can be lifted;
- puffiness under the eyes can be eliminated;
- bags under the eyes reduced;
- although not a cure for wrinkles, deeper wrinkles can also be reduced;
- fine facial lines can even be eliminated;
- double chins and jowls firmed up;
- age spots reduced, and even eliminated, depending on pre-existing conditions;
- blood and lymph circulation are improved by moisturizing the skin and returning an enviable glow to the face;
- collagen production is enhanced, which in turn brings on muscle tone and tightens the skin naturally;
- pores can be tightened so they appear smaller;
- restores hormonal imbalances to clear up acne and rosacea;
- all of which promote firmer, younger-looking skin.

As a non-invasive facial uplift, acupuncture has many benefits to recommend it. It's more affordable than costly cosmetic surgery, with hardly any facial disfigurement (such as swelling and discoloration) and is painless. Facial rejuvenation using acupuncture can literally take years off the face—while enhancing the body's overall health. Again, it's imperative to work with an experienced TCM practitioner with over a decade's worth of experience in this area.

Scientific notes. The *European Journal of Oriental Medicine*[83] reported a 1996 study by the *International Journal of Clinical Acupuncture* of 300 cases treated in China with cosmetic facial acupuncture. Ninety percent showed marked improvements after just one course of treatment.

---

[83] http://www.ejom.co.uk/vol-5-no-5/featured-articles/

Acupressure

History. Acupressure is also energy work pinpointing the meridians to unclog energy flow—but without needles. Pressure points are identified and worked on—for qi to revitalize and heal the body's blood and lymphatic flows in coursing through the meridians again.

Both blood and lymphatic systems play vital complementary roles. As noted, the liver cleanses the blood of toxins so the body's organs can receive nutrients. Through metabolic exchanges, waste products, such as carbon dioxide and cellular wastes, are excreted via the lymphatic system (or, the body's sewer system).

Benefits. There are twice as many lymph nodes as blood vessels in the body. Unlike the pumping heart, lymphatic fluid flows when chest muscles are activated during breathing. That's why acupressure practitioners advocate complementary modalities: 1) massage or *tuina*, 2) exercise which encourages deep breathing, such as qi gong or tai chi, 3) reducing stress and 4) body work massage so qi can flow optimally to restore the body's harmony.

Scientific notes. In TCM, the mantra for holistic body healing—reflected on face and skin—is, "Where qi goes, blood flows." That's how, according to Chinese medical precepts, beauty is expressed through healthy and nourishing blood—the river of life. More info on TCM is available at this U.S. National Institutes of Health website.[84]

FOOD AS MEDICINE

The ancient Chinese were also fastidious in honoring food as medicine (not unlike Hippocrates, "the father of modern medicine," in advocating this common sense dictum, as well.)

---

[84] http://nccam.nih.gov/health/chinesemed/

History. Step back a moment. Visualize how the ancient Chinese (and other ancient civilizations) had to live without refrigeration. It was vital to catch live food to slaughter, just before cooking for meals. This is still followed by old-timers in Chinatowns across North America, who gladly pay premium prices for fresh seafood, frog's legs, and poultry.

Benefits. Cooking and digesting food that has residual qi palpitating away makes a lot of sense in capturing maximum health benefits. In fact, the Chinese prize fresh coagulated blood (for cooking in soups) with herbs to nourish vital organs, to nourish glowing skin.

Foods were also dried in the sun for cooking later. We've promised you bird's nest and snow frog's fallopian tubes recipes. One of my medical assistants, Linda Huynh, got this recipe for birds' nest soup from her mother. Linda's mom also expertly prepares herbal teas to alleviate coughs and colds for family members. Linda says, "According to my mother, herbal teas can clear inner heat, toxins, soothe coughs, and rebalance the body's circulation."

BIRDS' NEST SOUP,
OR AN EXALTED DESSERT
(From Mrs. Huynh)

Cooking time: 2 hours and 30 minutes

2 oz. birds' nests (obtainable from Chinese pharmacies)
7-8 oz. crushed rock sugar
4 cups water

Soak birds' nests overnight. Remove feathers or other non-birds' nest items. Bring water to boil in a large pot. Simmer birds' nests for about 5 minutes; repeat this process twice. Rinse and squeeze dry the birds' nests. Place bird's nests in a pot and add 4 cups water. Bring to boil and simmer for 2 hours. Add rock sugar; stir to dissolve. Serve hot or warm.

<u>Benefits.</u> Stimulates cell growth, which helps skin rejuvenate with a radiant glow.

***

Linda also gave us a recipe for "Hasma snow frog fallopian tubes." An ancient beauty staple food of Chinese women, Hasma snow frogs (*rana chensinensis*, not regular frogs) are caught before or after the first snows in the northern provinces, such as Jinlin. According to Jacqueline M. Newman's[85] informative article, Hasma is moist, rich in hormones, and has a high lipid content—to lay healthy eggs come spring.

As this author recommends, the choicest Hasma "should look fatty, are glossy, have large sections, and look grainy with white membranes." Avoid them if they appear reddish-brown. Linda Huynh also got a recipe from Foodbuzz.com[86] for Hasma frog soup.

***

Hasma with Red Dates Sweet Soup

<u>Source:</u> http://www.foodbuzz.com/recipes/761471-hasma-with-red-dates-sweet-soup-

4 grams dried Hasma
10 pieces dried red dates
2 Tbsp rock sugar
2 cups water

Soak dried Hasma in cold water for about 4 hours or until it expands (to look like jelly.) Let it soak overnight in the fridge; then remove non Hasma items with a tweezer, picking out black or brown bits. Be gentle and don't break it up—leaving you a translucent jelly. Discard soaking water. De-seed 10 red dates. Boil cleaned Hasma and red dates with water and rock

---

[85] http://www.flavorandfortune.com/dataaccess/article.php?ID=248
[86] http://www.foodbuzz.com/recipes/761471-hasma-with-red-dates-sweet-soup-

sugar in a double-boiler for about 3 hours. When cooked, it becomes gelatinous and looks opaque.

Benefits. Protein-rich, high in hormones, Hasma rebalances a woman's hormonal needs and is also good for replenishing a woman's lipid and fat content—to impart a rosy, dewy glow to the skin.

Scientific notes. While research was not directly done on *rana chensinensis*, researchers at the University of Glasgow discovered a previously unreported discovery of similar protective protein cocktails designated as "ranaspumins."[87]

Acupuncturist and herbalist Joel Harvey Schreck, Ph.D., who goes by the pseudonym of Dr. Shen, has a simple glossary of centuries-old yin, yang, and neutral foods at: www.drshen.com/herbsforacne.htm. Scroll down to where he briefly discusses how skin inflammations develop as a result of body heat and dampness. That's where he suggests counter-balancing internal conditions with appropriate foods that are stimulating (yang), calming (yin), or neutral. Dr. Shen offers two caveats for lasting dietary changes:

1. Moderation is key, when altering your diet.

2. Changes and effects are more sustainable when introduced gradually.

That's why the Chinese consider food as medicine, as did Hippocrates. Ultimately, we are what we eat; and exercise is also important for healthy blood and lymph to circulate effectively.

---

[87] http://www.highbeam.com/doc/1G1-201328911.html?key=01-42160D517E1A146810080A16076F4B2E224E324D3417295C30420B61651B617F137019731B7B1D6B39

Mineral- and Animal-based Beauty Products

Linda Huynh has also used:

1. Pearl powder, and
2. Sheep's placenta.

Pearl Powder

Linda found pearl powder (sold as pellets) lightened her skin discolorations and gave her an overall "whitened complexion." As mentioned before, the most expensive form of pearl powder is ground from fresh-water pearls. Less expensive pearl powder is ground from oyster shells; worse, fillers such as chalk powder may also be used. Caveat emptor or buyers beware, do research first, before buying the wide varieties of online pearl powder products.

History. Pearl powder's extraordinary healing and beauty secrets have remained the prerogative of royalty—among the Chinese, Indian, Egyptian, and Mayan elites who could afford them.

- Benefits[88] include: A radiant and youthful complexion. With the body unable to manufacture collagen by age 40, pearl powder produces collagen, not only for skin, but also for healthy bones. Chinese empress Wu Zetian (625-705 ACE), who was the only female empress in Chinese history, astounded everyone when she ascended the throne at 65—with the radiant skin of a young woman. Of course, Empress Wu had the means to take pearl powder internally and applied it topically, too. It is also heart healthy and enhances immune support.

---

[88] http://www.pearlcium.com/ancient-stories.asp

- Improves blood circulation, while supporting healthy eyesight and mental acuity.
- Unlocks signal proteins for maximum absorption.

Scientific notes. In a double-bind crossover study, Dr. Rulin Xiu[89] found pearl powder to absorb nearly twice as well than calcium carbonate when taken with vitamin D. The pearl is also rich in "signal proteins" that control cellular growth. Signal proteins can:

- Stimulate new skin.
- Regenerate bone and increase bond density.
- Enhance skin tissue repair.

Sheep's Placenta

While not everyone's daily cream, Linda Huynh "felt fabulous" using sheep's placenta. It tightened, brightened, and hydrated her skin; plus "gave my skin a dewy look," she notes.

History. According to TCM records, the Chinese have been ingesting human placenta for 2,500 years for their rich proteins and nutrients. Placenta transports oxygen and nutrients from mother to fetus and is enriched with natural hormones.[90]

Benefits listed on the New Zealand Green Health website[91] include:

- Plumping, toning, and tightening skin.
- Normalizing pore size.
- "Exceptionally effective" for sun-damaged skin and age spots.

---

[89] http://www.pearlcium.com/the-pearl-secret.asp
[90] http://www.tcm-doctor.com/beauty/sheep_placenta_attraction.html
[91] http://www.nzgreenhealth.com/shop/product.php?id_product=22

• Stops oily, blemished, or loose skin.

<u>Scientific notes.</u> The FDA has strict requirements for certifying sheep's placenta as a dietary supplement, as a response from its Department of Health and Human Services shows.[92] Another source cautions that the FDA considers products with hormones as drugs—and should be certified before using it.[93]

By all accounts, please do research the latest beauty products first—before splurging on them. Satisfied customer testimonials and validated studies are surefire bets to try new, yet centuries-old, beauty products.

> *"Beautiful skin in not just genetic, but it is nurtured and requires effort. It is important not only to appreciate the beauty in others, but more important to understand your own and find the beauty that will radiate self-confidence and joy!"*
>
> —Yuan Ting, Actress, China

---

[92]

http://www.fda.gov/ohrms/dockets/dailys/03/feb03/020703/8004db33.pdf

[93] http://www.naturallycurly.com/curlreading/curl-products/sheeps-placenta-really

CHAPTER FIVE

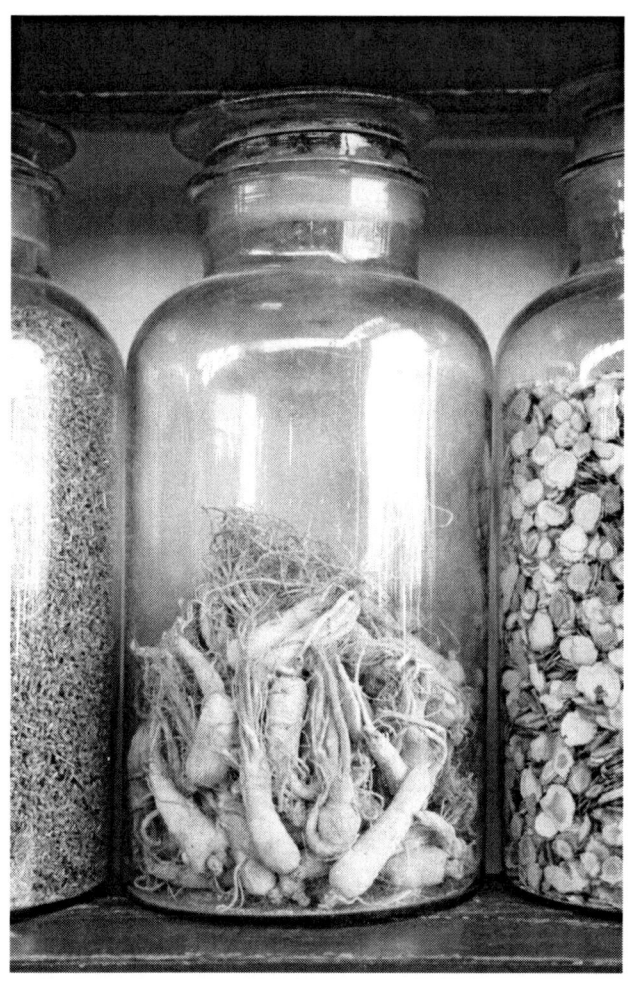

5

Why Asian Secrets Continue Impacting Beauty Treatments Today

At the YinOva Center, we take issue with the old adage that "beauty is only skin deep." Chinese medicine sees beauty as a reflection of the state of someone's whole body. Radiance comes from a strong, vibrant spirit, good nourishment, and enough rest. The holistic nature of Chinese medicine lends itself to the notion that beauty comes from within.

There is an old Chinese saying, "a woman's second face is in her hands," and Chinese women are meticulous about moisturizing and caring for their hands and feet. According to Chinese medicine, both the hands and the feet are microcosmic representations of the whole body. As our patients know, many of the most important acu-points are on the hands and feet, and stimulating these areas can have a beneficial effect on the whole body. Try to massage moisturizer into your hands and feet every day.[94]

—Jill Blakeway, M.S.L. Ac; Founder & Clinic
Director, YinOva Center

NEW YORK CITY ACUPUNCTURIST and Chinese herbalist Jill Blakeway emphasizes: "The holistic nature of Chinese medicine lends itself to the notion that beauty comes from within." For over 5,000 years, this ancient

---

[94] http://www.yinovacenter.com/blog/archives/1670/

beauty secret that has been at the cornerstone of Chinese Traditional Medicine is still the driving force for achieving radiant beauty today. Naturally. Thanks to Mother Nature's pharmacy of herbs and revitalizing life force energy—or qi. How amazing is this long and ancient history?

Jill tells me she uses TCM, or Traditional Chinese Medicine, to treat, "a broad range of issues." In fact, "Dermatology is a recognized specialty in Traditional Chinese Medicine. Treatments for skin disorders have been described as early as 1100-221 BCE in China. At our (YinOva) Center, we use acupuncture and Chinese herbs to treat acne, rosacea, dermatitis, psoriasis, eczema, alopecia, dry skin, and hives," Jill shares.[95]

(Apart from skin issues, Jill also treats—pain, allergies, digestive problems, gynecological problems, and migraine—with acupuncture and herbs.)

TCM for Treating Eczema

In using TCM for treating eczema, Jill Blakeway advocates:

- Strengthening the immune system. When the body is able to resist non-stop onslaughts from pathogens (bacteria, virus, stress, pollution, etc.), this decreases sensitivity and vulnerability to external environmental hazards.

- Balancing the internal organ systems. By addressing internal imbalances contributing to, or causing, eczema, a patient can heal from within. Jill explains the liver is important in supplying clean blood to organs, by carrying nutrients and oxygen to body cells, and toxic wastes away from them. However, a sluggish liver would be less efficient in carrying out

---

[95] Email received on 3/7/2011.

these functions, with the blood overburdened by excess toxins. When this happens, the liver depends on the skin to "push" out toxins—resulting in rashes. That's why it's imperative to maintain the liver's internal harmony.

- <u>Releasing toxins from the skin.</u> When toxic pus builds up, itchy postules form on the skin. Herb-based topical creams (such as green tea paste) help dry out and eliminate these uncomfortable and disfiguring red rashes.

- <u>Building the yin and blood.</u> The body is a holistic combination of yang (hot, dynamic) and yin (cool, moisturizing) complementary forces. When in harmony, the forces of yin and yang are operating optimally and reflected in the body's good health. However, as we age, moisturizing yin energy also diminishes—manifesting as drier and duller-looking skin. Luckily, this situation can be remedied with nourishing and repairing damaged skin by using herbs from nature's pharmacy, such as schizandra. A beauty tonic, schizandra is considered a youth-preserving herb that promotes skin suppleness and smoothness, and in re-moisturizing it.

Jill also mentions reishi mushroom in her blog, "5 Chinese Beauty Secrets."[96] A versatile adaptogen, reishi mushrooms regenerate the liver, oxygenate blood, calm the mind, and balance blood sugar.

Yet another historic herb Jill lists in this article is astragalus, a sweet-tasting herb. A major tonic herb in TCM, astragalus builds immunity, balances body fluids, lowers blood pressure, and increases stamina. She notes, too, that modern research shows astragalus increases the production of

---

[96] http://www.yinovacenter.com/blog/archives/1670/

white blood cells—the body's first line of defense in fighting
infection.

TCM for Treating Teenage Acne

Jill Blakeway's TCM analysis of teenage acne and how to
treat it is worth noting. In *Treating Teenage Acne with Chinese
Herbs*,[97] she cites two conditions: "heat" and "dampness."
Both can be caused by internal and external factors and can
be corrected naturally to rebalance homeostasis.

"Heat." In a teenage body bursting with hormonal
changes, getting the "zits" is devastating for an age group
that's pretty self-conscious of its image. While yang or
dynamic heat is needed to propel the body's activities, too
much of a good thing can cause zits to pop. Internal reasons
range from: 1) emotional (such as peer pressure) and the
inability to talk things out and to release them; 2) hormonal
imbalances; and 3) "deficient blood" or nutritional
deficiencies with the teen not eating nutritionally-sound meals
while trying to get by on fast foods and greasy hamburgers. In
TCM, deficient blood is full of toxins trying to "push" out
through acne-riddled skin. External causes of heat include
chemicals on the skin, too much physical exertion or extra-
curricular active sports and/or over-stimulating foods, such
as deep-fried, oily foods.

"Dampness." The body's yin or moisturizing element
can become too damp. When excess moisture builds up in
tissues, bacteria and yeast begin to thrive—thus forming
pustules or cystic acne. Another internal cause is a faulty
digestive system—further stressed out by irregular eating
habits and a diet heavy on fatty and greasy foods that teens
find easy to fall into.

At the YinOva Center, acupuncture is used to clear acne
and other forms of skin inflammation, while herbs are used

---

[97] http://www.yinovacenter.com/blog/archives/3010/

to treat dampness and heat. Herbal concoctions are customized to address each patient's unique underlying causes.

Herbs heal naturally because patients take them in the original form. However, modern medicines are generally synthesized to mimic active plant extracts—with the added problem that synthesized medicines can induce more side effects.

As Jill explains, eastern medicine emphasizes prevention of diseases by focusing on:

1. moving qi and blood as they need to flow through the meridians,

2. protecting the body from accumulating toxic wastes,

3. "clearing damp accumulation," otherwise known as getting rid of excess fat cells, and

4. supporting the body's natural defenses with enhanced immunity from the constant barrage of pathogens.

Jill points out, "Western and Eastern medicine may come from a different frame of reference, but their findings are very similar. The advice we give is, therefore, not inconsistent, whether you see the world in an Eastern or a Western way. (As you know, at The YinOva Center, we do a bit of both.)"[98]

The power of natural healing from herbs and re-balancing qi to flow efficiently again along the meridians with acupuncture are two powerful testaments of how simple and easy the body's health and skin issues can be maintained and healed from within.

The bonus? A highly visible radiant state of good health—and a glowing skin complexion that mirrors a person's internal harmony and well-being.

---

[98] http://www.yinovacenter.com/blog/archives/388/

This is the simple secret of ancient Asian beauty secrets—that *anyone* can access and use to maintain their own states of beauty and health for lifelong enjoyment, good looks, and happiness.

Herbs for Beautiful Skin

I asked Jill Blakeway about herbs promoting beautiful skin. She suggests[99]:

1. *Hu ma ren* or sesame seeds to moisten dry skin. In his book, *Healing with Whole Foods* (3rd edition), Paul Pitchford explains that sesame "lubricates *dryness*, working as an emollient when applied to dry and cracked skin; it also relieves constipation. Sesame oil also detoxifies. It destroys ringworm, scabies, and most fungal skin diseases. It is a superior massage oil for sore muscles and the pain of rheumatism/ arthritis."[100]

2. *Ku shen* or sophora treats inflamed, itchy skin.

3. *Shi gao* or gypsum is very cooling and great for treating acne.

4. *Zhen zhu mu,* or mother-of-pearl shell, heals skin blemishes.

5. *Shu di huang* (prepared rehmannia root) treats dry skin and rashes.

6. *Jin yin hua,* or honeysuckle flower, treats redness— especially around the eyes.

7. *Xuan shen* (scrophularia root) treats eczema and itching.

---

[99] Email received on 3/7/2011.
[100] Page 185.

8. *Jing jie* (schizonepeta herb) treats rashes and dermatitis.

Dr. Barbara Custer of Mill Valley, California, says wild yam extract helps teens with cystic acne, while white ginseng is good for women's skin.

Herbs for Overall Good Health

Additionally, Jill Blakeway's "7 Chinese Herbs" for good health are:

1. *Dang shen*, Radix Codonopsis Pilosulae, is a qi tonic and immune booster.

2. *Bai zhu*, Rhizoma Atractylodis Macrocephalae, is a qi tonic that also supports the digestive system.

3. *Fu ling*, Sclerotium Poriae Cocos, is mildly diuretic and improves liver function.

4. *Dang gui* root or Radix Angelicae Sinensis is a blood tonic often used to treat gynecological problems, such as irregular menses.

5. *Bai shao* or Radix Paeoniae Lactiflorae is a blood tonic that also helps with liver function.

6. *Chuan xiong*, Rhizoma Ligustici Chuanxiong, promotes circulation.

7. *Shu di huang*, Radix Rehmanniae Preparata, is a yin tonic that moistens dryness.

Other TCM Applications for Health & Beauty

Over the course of thousands of years, other TCM healing modalities have been honed and proved their efficacies, such as:

1. <u>Cupping.</u> A Korean friend, Yumi Kim and owner of Curtain Call, says, "I get frozen shoulder from using

the computer often. I tried massage and physical therapies, but came away impressed with cupping. Cupping initially caused dark bruises, but eventually disappeared; and my shoulder feels so much better now." Cupping is a method of applying heat therapy to unclog meridians for qi to flow again. When qi and blood circulate unimpeded, the body's internal harmony is resuscitated by body cells receiving oxygen and nutrients from the blood.

2. Moxibustion is another form of TCM heat therapy. Alice Lee, senior beauty editor at Beijing Raylie Magazine House, tells me that moxibustion therapy is huge in China's larger cities, such as Beijing and Shanghai. "Moxa" is made from rolled mugwort herb, cigar-like, and burned over acupuncture points to unclog meridians. True to flow, when qi and blood are unobstructed, internal harmony is maintained. Moxibustion is used for preventive and curative measures—and popular in spas and beauty salons, Alice says.

3. Food Therapy. As is pretty obvious by now, food therapy is popular and practical in maintaining beauty and the joy it gifts diners. Dr. Song Ping, a dermatologist in China, says, ""Rose, honey, and milk are good for pale complexions. Green tea and bitter gourd are good for acne." Dr. Ping also suggests cold green tea to cool and calm down sensitive and inflamed skin. She says red wine and ginseng masks are commonly used in China, Korea, and Japan. Be it bird's nest soup, Hasma frog fallopian tubes, or rich green tea, connoisseurs of the fine life and beautiful living enjoy Mother Nature's abundance—while feeling and looking good.

It's appropriate to end this chapter on how Far Eastern healing and beauty modalities are now going global—even as the western arrow is making its mark in Korea, Japan, and China with botox injections, double eyelid surgery, and fractional laser resurfacing to polish and brighten skin.

New York City beautician Mary Schook, known as the "Beauty Engineer," looks to Asia for advanced beauty treatments for her clients. Paradoxically, the majority of her clients are from Hong Kong and Korea. She says, "Their major concern is keeping their skin as clean and bright as possible." She uses a serum-based micro-dermabrasion, followed by LED (light-emitting diode) skin treatments. Interestingly, NASA first developed LED treatments in the 1970s to help astronauts heal faster during space travel. Today, these hand-held devices can be used at home for acne and other blemishes. LEDs are even touted to be anti-aging.

The next chapter discusses skin issues specific to Asians. Not exactly peaches-and-cream, the composition of Asian skin is quite different form Caucasian skin—and merits its own discourse on prevalent issues and relevant treatments.

The Yellow Emperor said:
"Yin/Yang are the way of Heaven and Earth,
the great principle and outline of everything,
the parents of change,
the root and source of life and death,
the palace of gods.
Treatment of disease should be based
Upon the roots of Yin/Yang."
--Nei Jing (First Century, B.C.E.)

From: *The Encyclopedia of Chinese Medicine*
Dr. Duo Gao, Editor (Carlton Books. 1997)

CHAPTER SIX

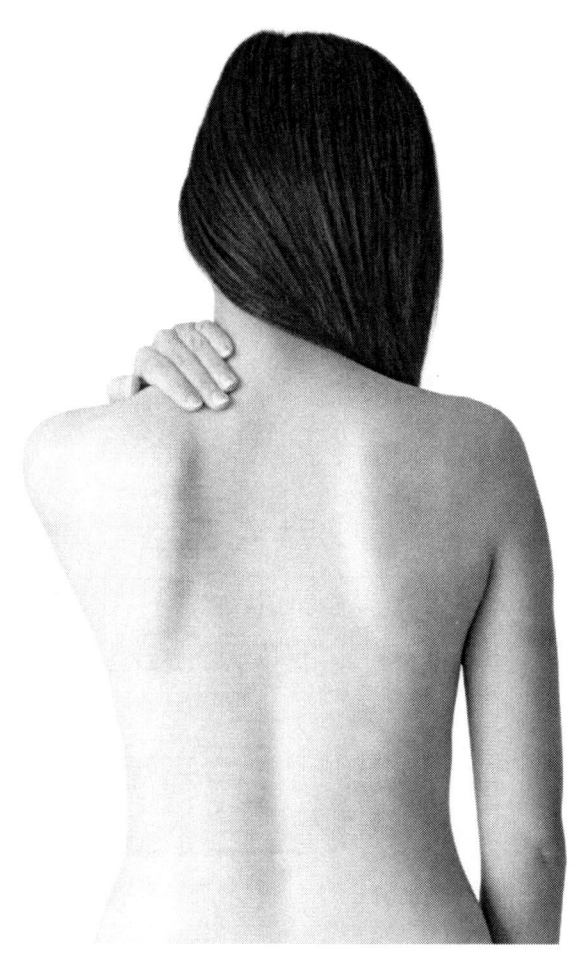

6

Common Asian Skin Issues

Acne in Asian skin can be a terrible problem. When Asians get acne, it tends to be more severe and inflammatory, with painful red bumps and pustules on the skin, versus non-inflammatory acne with whiteheads and blackheads. Action needs to be taken immediately and aggressively—otherwise, the acne can lead to scarring and hyperpigmentation. Because Asian skin tends to get more inflammatory acne and can lead to discoloration and dark spots, as well as scarring, it is important to seek a doctor to treat the acne aggressively and to shorten the duration of the outbreak.

—Marie Jhin, M.D.

A S I NOTE ABOVE, the genetic makeup of Asian skin is quite different from Caucasian skin, which, therefore, produces vastly different skin conditions and issues, such as:

1. Melanocytes or pigment cells in Asian skin produce more abundant amounts of eumelanin than pheomelanin (which are more plentiful in Caucasian skin). This means Asian skin generally tans better for a darker skin—which also helps protect the skin a little better than lighter skin.

2. Melanocytes in Asian skin produce granules called melanosomes that are larger and more spread out than in fairer skin (where they are smaller and more

93

dense). This, too, gives East Asians a darker skin color that we see.

3. Melanocytes in darker skin are much more active as they produce more pigment than in whiter skin. However, although more pigment gives Asian skin more sun protection, it can also be more problematic with skin pigmentation and irregularities.

4. In Asian skin, the collagen bundle that makes skin firm and full is bundled together more thickly. This can be beneficial in giving Asian skin less wrinkles; however, it may lead to other issues, such as scar formation or keloid scar formation.

8 COMMON ASIAN SKIN ISSUES

Some common Asian skin issues I see in my patients include the following.

1. <u>Melasma</u> is very common among Asian women. Also called cholasma or "the mask of pregnancy," melasma can pop up in men and women (even when not pregnant). Hormones, genetics, and sun exposure appear to play a role in causing melasma. These brown patches are usually found on the cheek, forehead, and upper lip. Melasma is especially devastating if it has a deep component because it's then harder to treat.

   The most important first step is prevention—by using sun block every day, because the sun aggravates melasma. Sometimes, melasma fades post-pregnancy, or when hormonal activities from birth control pills are stopped. But, even then, melasma can continue to form.

   First-line treatment for melasma includes sun block and topical lightening creams. I like Obagi Nuderm® and Glytone Clarifying Kit®. Triluma® can also be used if the melasma is located in a small area. Depending on the patient's condition, I also use chemical peels or Cosmelan® melasma masks.

A Korean Board certified dermatologist, Hyeonsook Lee, M.D., also prescribes glycolic and amino acid peels, iontophoresis, and hydroquinone creams. She iterates, "As you know, melasma is difficult to cure and relapses are common. I like to emphasize to patients they avoid sun exposure and sleep well."[101]

2. <u>Postinflammatory hyperpigmentation (PIH)</u> appears after trauma has been inflicted on skin, such as after a burn, acne eruptions, or even a laser treatment gone bad. PIH is particularly common in darker ethnic skin. Again, solar exposure exacerbates PIH. Fading creams, such as hydroquinones, would block further skin pigmentation. A dermatologist can also prescribe cortisone or retinoid creams to clear up pigmentation. Avoiding trauma is obviously important, but treating it quickly is also important, using creams such as Avene's Cicalfate® and Biafine cream, which helps wounds heal faster without leaving a discoloration. Once dark marks are formed, I like to use a 4% hydroquinone cream like Epiquin Microgel®.

3. <u>Acne</u> in Asians is more severe and inflammatory with painful red bumps and pustules and, therefore, needs to be treated immediately and aggressively. Otherwise, it can lead to scarring and PIH. There are many causes for acne, including over-active oil glands producing more acne bacteria. Less inflammatory acne would result in whiteheads and blackheads.

---

[101] Email received on 2/27/2011.

To alleviate acne, use "non-comedogenic" cleansers, sun blocks, and cosmetics. People think that using more and thicker makeup would cover up the condition—while, in fact, it becomes a vicious cycle because the pores become clogged. I advise them to use mineral makeup instead, which is composed of micro, nano-sized particles which enable makeup to be absorbed easily.

Although dirty skin and not washing the face do not contribute to acne, it's still very important to keep the face clean by removing facial oil. Keeping the skin clean also helps topical medications penetrate and work better in clearing up acne. I recommend gentle cleansers such as Cetaphil®, Neutrogena Clear-Pore Wash®, or Cereve Cleanser®.

Toners are also helpful in removing oil and prepping the skin for medication. For Asians without sensitive skin, toners such as Aquaglycolic® or Obagi® are helpful. Avoid toners with alcohol as the first ingredient.

Alpha and beta hydroxy products have been used for centuries. They are natural acids found in plants and foods, such as sugarcane and milk, which can unplug clogged pores, improve texture, and even out skin tone. These products are found in cleansers, moisturizers, toners, and peels. I recommend Aqua glycolic cleanser by Merz; Vivite cleanser and Neutrogena Oil Free Acne Wash are cleansers that are for oilier skin.

In Asian skin, I would start with the lowest percentage of alpha hydroxy, such as glycolic acid or lactic acid, because the acids can cause dryness and mild irritation. A beta hydroxy acid, such as salicylic acid, can be helpful but, again, start at the lowest percentage as advised by a doctor.

If over-the-counter products don't work, I suggest seeking a dermatologist right away. Although there are no magic pills, the doctor can prescribe oral antibiotics to decrease inflammation and reduce acne bacteria. They can also recommend Accutane, a strong dose of Vitamin A that is very effective for severe acne. The doctor can also recommend topical prescription creams that may be higher in concentration than over-the-counter medications. The doctor can also recommend topical prescription creams that may be higher in concentration than over-the-counter medications, such as Differin cream or lotion, Epiduo, Aczone, Veltin, or Atralin.

A word of caution: Asians get easily irritated from Benzoyl peroxide and retinoids (topical Vitamin A creams). Many confuse the redness and dryness that may develop from using these products as an allergy—when, in fact, it is a mild irritation. I find Asian patients can continue using these products, but in smaller amounts, in gradually introducing them, or mixing them with a mild moisturizer. Retinols that are milder can be used, such as Avene's Retinal cream, La Roche-Posay Biomedic Retinol cream, Neutrogena Healthy Skin Visibly Even Night Concentrate, and Kinerase Protherapy Retin A.

Chemical peels may be an effective treatment for acne. These peels are usually done at the doctor's office. I recommend a beta hydroxy or salicylic acid peel.

However, it is important to start at a lower strength since these peels can cause irritation and more peeling in Asian skin. Patients would need to stop applying retinoids three days prior to the peel treatment.

Cortisone injections can be very helpful to reduce inflammation quickly, plus prevent scarring and hyperpigmentation. The injections are done at the doctor's clinic and supplementary to other treatments. Usually, if done correctly, acne pimples will go away in a few days. This should not be the only treatment for acne—but it is useful, especially if there is inflammatory acne and you have a special event coming up and want to look good.

Lasers and light devices are becoming more popular for treating acne. Heat from the laser helps shrink oil glands, thus decreasing oil production and bacteria formation. I find these treatments useful if the person cannot tolerate oral or topical treatments. However, these treatments require multiple sessions and are more costly.

Light treatments also work by reducing acne bacteria buildup. There are many devices; again, these treatments have to be done in multiple sessions and may not eliminate acne completely.

Photodynamic therapy with Levulan is FDA-approved to treat pre-cancerous lesions and is also used to treat acne. Levulan has been found to shrink oil or sebaceous glands and to reduce oil accumulations. This treatment can be effective, but requires avoiding exposure to sun or light sources for two days after treatment.

Avoid picking at the skin or scubbing it—and be patient. These products do take time to work, but can make a huge difference in preventing permanent scarring.

4. <u>Atopic dermatitis or eczema</u> is very common among Asians. I see this in my clinic often, from infants to adults. Usually infants have it on the face and body, while adults are more likely to have it on their hands. Eczema can be genetic; patients can also have

asthma and allergies—or all three at the same time. Eczema can be triggered by irritating products, allergies to food, or emotional stress; and it is a disease that becomes a vicious cycle of itch and scratch. The skin becomes crusty, very dry, and scaly, even dark and thick. Often, the rash gets infected from open wounds that come from scratching.

Naoko Tani-Fukuchi tells me, "I suffered from atopic dermatitis for many years. Finally, I found a Korean herbal soap that helped immensely, and a Japanese green tea peeling gel. The soap also removed skin blemishes and wrinkles. I've also heard it helps to moisturize aging skin as it helps to alleviate itching that comes from dry skin."[102]

There are many treatments for eczema. The key is to control the itch and to not scratch, in containing a vicious cycle. This can be accomplished by taking antihistamines, wearing gloves, or clipping fingernails to minimize scratch marks. It is important to keep the skin cool, not too hot, and to moisturize it regularly. I also tell patients to avoid anything that makes them itch—such as itchy clothing, over-drying skin, or environmental causes, such as dust mites and chemicals. It is very important to know that **stress can make eczema worse.**

Sometimes, discovering the trigger takes detective work. My oldest daughter had atopic dermatitis along dry, scaly patches; she also developed very red, round inflamed patches symmetrically on both posterior thighs during her first grade. As a dermatologist and mother, I treated her with the best medications.

However, the symptoms would go away—only to return more "angry." This went on for a few

---

[102] Email received on 2/20/2011.

months. One day, I went to her school and sat on her little chair. That's when it clicked! I noticed two shiny screws on her chair—and realized she had an allergy to nickel, a metal alloy. I made her a fitted cushion for her chair. Voila! Her rash went away.

In terms of treatments for eczema, I recommend a topical steroid cream for the flares, as well as moisturizers and avoiding triggers. Antihistamines and non-steroidal prescription creams are also helpful. And, I recommend a bath with a cup of bleach at least once a month to prevent bacterial infections from forming. Swimming in chlorinated water is okay. This may be a life-long problem and needs to be carefully monitored under a doctor's care. I also recommend Cereve® cleanser or moisturizer, Aquaphor®, Dove® soap, Avene® Trixera moisturizer, Aveeno® oatmeal baths, and Neutrogena® Tsal shampoo and DHS® clear shampoo.

5. Keratosis pilaris are small multiple bumps usually appearing on upper arms, sometimes on legs, the back, or face. These small bumps are hair follicles filled by dry plugs. This can be genetic and occur more commonly in those with allergies or eczema. It is more common during the cold winter months. People try to scrub the bumps away, but this can be irritating and make the bumps worse.

   I recommend a skin softening lotion, such as Amlactin® or alpha beta hydroxy acids, or Glytone's KP® Kit. Gentle cleaning helps, but not aggressive exfoliation. Chemical peels administered by a dermatologist are also helpful.

6. Seborrheic keratoses are superficial and benign growths commonly found in areas exposed to the

100

sun—on the face, neck, and arms. They are common among Asians who are predisposed genetically, or can occur post-pregnancy and among older people. These multiple bumps of various sizes look like they have been "stuck on," almost as if they can be scratched off.

When my father, an avid golfer, comes to visit, his only request is to remove the brown bumps from his face. A dermatologist removes them with liquid nitrogen, or uses a hyfercator to burn them off, which leaves very little scarring.

7. Keloids or hypertrophic scars are unlike regular scars. They are raised and often very disfiguring scars from any type of trauma—even ear-piercing or from an acne scar. It is not known why some people are more prone to keloids, but again, it can be hereditary. The skin for some reason develops thick collagen fibers that create large irregular scars.

    A Chinese friend, Amy Chu, has problems with keloid scarring. "I do keloid easily. It's so annoying. I have two huge keloids on my shoulder blades, which I think started off as pimples many years ago," Amy says.

    I developed a hypertrophic scar on my arm from an immunization shot I received as a child. As a teenager, I remember feeling self-conscious in not wanting to wear sleeveless shirts. The good news is—there are treatments that can help make scars less visible. The scars, though, may never completely heal.

    Treatments include steroid injections, removing the scar, and injecting steroid injections to prevent it from re-enlarging. Occasionally, other injections can be given such as 5-FU, a chemotherapy medicine. Topically, an immuno-modulator, such as Imiquimoid cream can be used, as well as silicone sheets and applying pressure to the scars. Laser treatments can reduce the redness, such as a pulse-dye laser.

8. Sun damage from solar exposure. Unlike Caucasian patients more concerned with wrinkles and fine lines, my Asian patients worry about age or brown spots. The most important advice I can offer is to use sunscreen lotions higher than SPF 30. I like Elta®, Anthelios®, Burnout®, Neutrogena® Helioplex sun blocks.

Treatments for sun-damaged brown spots include trying over-the-counter products first, such as Shisedo White Lucent Concentrated Brightening Serum, Neostrata Skin Brightening gel, Cellex-C Fade Away gel, and Clinique Acne Solutions.

If that doesn't work, treatments and products in the dermatologist office should be sought, which include: the NY:Yag laser, Intense Pulse Light (IPL), bleaching creams, such as hydroquinones, and acids, such as azealic, kojic, and mandelic. Chemical peels and microdermabrasion are also effective in removing sun spots and healing sun-damaged skin.

Like other Chinese women in their mid-40s, New Yorker Vera Sung finds, "Our biggest skin issue has to be age spots that suddenly appear on our faces. The big question is whether to treat them with fading creams or to go for laser treatments. And how to prevent more from appearing by staying out of the sun, using sun screens and more fading creams."[103]

Patients ask me if Asians have more sensitive skin. I notice Asian skin is more sensitive to products, such as benzoyl peroxides and retinoid creams prescribed for acne and wrinkles. Skin starts getting red and scaly with retinoid cream, and

---

[103] Email received on 2/20/2011.

patients wonder if they are allergic. I reassure them they are not allergic—it's just that they have to gradually introduce their skin to the product.

In the following chapter, we'll discuss some unconventional cosmetic treatments currently *en vogue* in the Far East. Think botox for filling in wrinkles? Well, think botox for softening square jaw lines, too—an idea that's popular with many Asian women in China, Japan, and Korea.

CHAPTER SEVEN

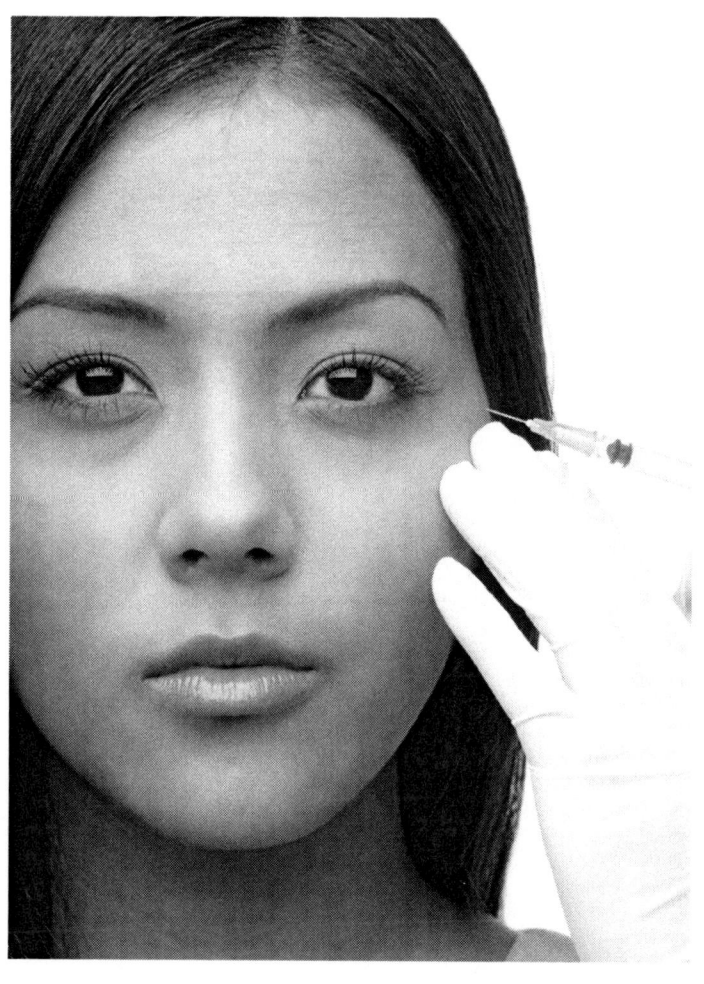

7

Modern Asian Beauty Tips, Treatments, & Trends

Today's modern Chinese woman continues to prefer flawless skin. That's why whitening products are so popular in China. Chinese women are fighting their yellow skin tone, and use a lot of anti-spot or brightening products. Also, IPL (Intense Pulse Light) is hot in China.

Chinese women want to look slim, slim, slim! Slimming products and treatments are bestsellers for body care, because we think the body's lovely curves are great to show off sexy glamour.

I also think the trend is to get "ageless skin" without the pain—for products and non-invasive treatments. Digitally delivered beauty information via special mobile apps for iPhones and iPads will also play important roles in updating Chinese women on the latest beauty care and products.

—Ms. Huang Ting, China Cosmo Deputy Beauty Editor

LET'S FORWARD WIND NOW from discussing ancient Asian beauty secrets to see what some of the latest prevailing beauty trends are in China, Japan, and Korea today:

- What changes do we discern, and what ancient secrets are still thriving?

- What are appropriate cosmetic treatments for Asians?

- What are some unconventional treatments, and have they gone too far?

In my clinic in the San Francisco Bay Area, the most popular treatments for my Asian patients include: Intense Pulse Light (IPL), Silkpeel® microinfusion, Botox®, Dysport®, fillers such as Restylane®, Juviderm®, Radiesse® and a skin-tightening procedure, such as Thermage®.

What about the Far East?

As *China Cosmo*'s deputy beauty editor, Huang Ting has her pulse on the latest beauty trends in her country. She's honest in pointing out how Chinese women are still fighting their yellow skin tones—and continuing with the age-old classic beauty ideal of whitening their skin in trying to appear attractive.

Now, more than ever, it's also inevitable for modern science and technology to come to the rescue of those seeking resolutions for their irritating skin problems. What's happening today in the Far East so we may learn what, and how, to adapt these ideas on a larger scale?

Modern Technology and Asian Aesthetics

First, let's examine some technological breakthroughs serving the science of beauty currently gaining popular in China, Korea, and Japan. As Huang Ti points out above, Chinese women are looking forward to "ageless skin" without the pain—with non-invasive high-tech and electronic tools gaining popularity.

1. <u>IPL or Intense Pulse Light</u> is commonly used to remove sun-damaged skin and age, brown or sun spots (also known as sun-induced freckles). Painless, gentle, quick (it's all over in about 10 minutes for each session) and non-invasive, IPL is the technique of choice as a skin brightening treatment for the

majority of Chinese men and women, *Cosmo China*'s deputy beauty editor Haung Ting reports.[104]

IPL is very popular around the world, too, because it efficiently reverses photo-damaged skin for a more youthful, luminous look. The face, hands, and body all benefit from IPL treatments, which consist of four to six sessions at three-week intervals. Broad-spectrum light is held over sun-damaged skin and penetrates through the damaged cells and tissues. The body naturally removes the damaged tissues via the blood stream. IPL also removes facial hair, varicose veins, and tattoos.

2. <u>Intracel laser</u> treatment is currently making a huge impact in Korean plastic surgery. This innovative technique combines modern science with acupuncture by reaching deeper into the dermis for more lasting collagen production and overall skin rejuvenation.

   Based on "FRM" or "Fractional Radiofrequency Microneedling," cells are reported to have developed fibroblasts faster according to a June 2010 study conducted by Un-Cheol Yeo, M.D.[105] This study found microneedles left minimal damage on the epidermis and upper dermis, the top two layers of the skin. FRM impacted the lower dermis on a deeper level with dermal heating conducive to producing fibroblasts. Dr. Yeo's study concluded FRM is suitable for tightening skin, reducing wrinkles, and treating scars.

   (Note: As the U.S. National Institutes of Health explains, when cells are hurt or damaged, myofibroblasts in the skin produce collagen to help

---

[104] Email received on 3/13/2011.
[105] http://intracel.blogspot.com/

healing—thereby producing new skin that's firm and smooth.[106])

3. Referred to as "skin toning," the <u>Nd:YAG laser</u>, with longer light wavelengths, is more effective in penetrating through the dermis (or skin). Dr. Takahiro Fujimoto, M.D., Ph.D., of Tokyo University's 2005 White Paper on "Non-ablative Skin Rejuvenation utilizing a combination of Q-switched and long-pulse Nd:YAG laser"[107] found that after eight months, patients "reported improvement in skin texture, pore size, fine wrinkles, and spotty pigments." Currently, the Q-switched Nd:YAG laser is a safe and popular laser treatment for improving skin texture and, especially, pore size reduction.

My Korean colleague Dr. Hyung-Gi Cha says doctors there successfully treat melasma, freckles, lentigo, and seborrheic keratosis with this form of "laser toning."[108] Dr. Cha also points out the previous laser method, FRM, is effective for acne scars, large pores, and wrinkles.

4. <u>Bleaching.</u> Another Korean colleague, Dr. Hyeonsook Lee, uses bleaching agents, such as chemical peels (glycolic and amino acids), iontophoresis, and hydroquinone to treat melasma. She knows Korean dermatologists also prescribe: tranexamic acid, multi-vitamins, and placenta extract.[109]

---

[106] http://www.ncbi.nlm.nih.gov/books/NBK26889/

[107] http://www.lutronic.com/en/documents/White_Paper_Fujimoto_Poresize_Reduction_with_Spectra_Peel_w_photos(white_paper).pdf

[108] Email received on 2/23/2011.

[109] Email received on 2/27/2011.

5. Botox injections, while getting more popular, are still suspect in China, Huang Ting notes. However, in Korea and Japan, botox injections are gaining big strides in helping women reclaim their self-esteem in different ways. While Western women use botox to erase wrinkles, Asian women use botox for entirely different reasons—to soften square jaw lines by filling them out and to atrophy cheek muscles in shrinking an all too-round facial landscape.

6. Fat-dissolving injections. Dr. Hyeonsook Lee has success in using PPC or "phophatidylcholine." Other fat-dissolving agents she mentions are: a) aminophillin, b) HPL or hypotonic pharmacologic lipodissolution, and c) LLD or lypolytic lymphatic drainage.[110] She also points out that liposuction is far and away more effective in removing body fat.

7. Plastic surgery. *Time* magazine reports, "Dr. Suh In Seock, a surgeon in Seoul, has struggled to find the best way to fix an affliction the Koreans call *muu-dari* and the Japanese call *daikon-ashi*: radish-shaped calves. Liposuction, so effective on the legs of plump Westerners, doesn't work on Asians since muscle, not fat, accounts for the bulk."[111] Dr. Suh explains he discovered how severing a nerve behind the knee atrophies the muscle—and reduces calf size by up to 40 percent.

This same article also reports Asian men taking advantage of surgical procedures to regain their self-worth. Tokyo plastic surgeon Dr. Katsuya Takasu looks 10 years younger than his 57 years. His beauty secrets? Face lifts and chemical peels. Dr. Takasu has had eyelid surgery (blepharoplasty) and jaw surgery. He tells *Time* magazine reporter Lisa Takeuchi

---

[110] Email received on 2/27/2011.
[111] http://www.time.com/time/world/article/0,8599,2047454,00.html

Cullen, "I had a colleague insert a golden wire in my chin to prevent sagging." He observes, "Men are uptight about seeming too vain. But it's true that when you look old, you're treated that way."

More so than women, this *Time* magazine feature notes that men are taking to plastic surgery to advance their careers. Taiwanese comedian Tsai Tou was once known as "the ugliest man in show business." He so desired professional advancement in hosting his own talk show that he: 1) had eyelid surgery, 2) removed the bags under his eyes, 3) heightened his nose, and 4) flattened his wrinkles with botox. Now highly successful with a "trustworthy" look preferred by TV viewers, Tsai Tou was driven by economic necessity, not vanity, in seeking plastic interventions.

Taiwanese entertainer Ching Wei is now an award-winning media personality after spending $60,000 on plastic surgery. "It's a miracle. Everything you see about me is the work of plastic surgery—my facial skin, implanted hair, and restored retina," he says in this *Time* article.

The repertoire for cosmetic enhancements has certainly increased from ancient times, hasn't it? A noteworthy trend now happening in China is, "going back to using Chinese medicine and herbal ingredients," says Huang Ting, *Cosmo China*'s deputy beauty editor. She adds that natural and organic beauty products are getting more popular because of safety concerns that beauty products might be using ingredients that are not as advertised.[112]

---

[112] Email received on 3/13/2011.

Ancient Asian Beauty Secrets are Alive and Well Today!

Not only in China is the beauty cycle coming full circle in returning to traditional herbal products and medicinal techniques. As noted, Japanese women and men are also returning to their traditional beauty roots in using ingredients from the plant and animal kingdoms. In Korea, forward-moving cosmetics companies, such as Amore Pacific, are super-charging cosmetics using high-quality ginseng and bamboo sap (or "divine water" as the ancients called it) with nano-technology in fashioning beauty products more easily absorbed by body cells.

It's worth noting, too, that in the collective aspirations of women (and men) everywhere seeking only the best skin care products, upscale American department stores, such as Neiman Marcus and Bergdorf Goodman, are now carrying Amore Pacific's Sulwhasoo cosmetics because these products are entirely herbal-based—and that they had not seen skin care products of this nature before.[113]

Alice Lee, senior beauty editor at Beijing Raylie Magazine House, says plant-based cosmetics by local companies, such as Herborist, are popular in China.[114]

On its website, Herborist[115] explains their products are based on:

- the ancient healing powers of plants;
- balancing the energies of plants and humans fundamental to the longevity and well-being of all living organisms; and
- enabling everyone to live serene and harmonious lives.

---

[113] http://blog.bergdorfgoodman.com/womens-style/sulwhasoo
[114] Email received on 2/19/2011.
[115] http://www.herborist-international.com/brand/traditional-chinese-medecine

"Inner beauty and visible beauty nurture each other," this Web site advises. It notes that in 2800 B.C.E., Emperor Shennong studied 365 plants and compiled the *Ben Cao Jing* to describe how plants release energies for healing. This classic remains an authoritative source on Chinese herbal sciences today.

According to Alice Lee, the three top fashionable trends in China today are: 1) Botox® treatments, 2) hyaluronic acid injections, and 3) IPL or Intense Pulse Light to correct photo-damaged and every kind of blemished skin. (As an aside, hyaluronic acids such as Juviderm® and Restylane® draw in water to plump up and fill in lines and wrinkles—in giving skin a firm, fresh, dewy, and youthful look.)

Alice also says moxibustion is now offered as a beauty treatment in Chinese spas and beauty salons. ("Moxa" continues to be a common medical treatment in Chinese hospitals, as well.) A form of heat therapy that's similar in principle to cupping, "moxa" uses heat to release clogged meridians for qi (the body's life force) and blood streams to flow unobstructed again. Once the body's qi, blood, and lymph systems are reinvigorated, natural defenses are shored up—a healing concept at the cornerstone of TCM (Traditional Chinese Medicine). Alice says additional benefits of moxibustion include: stress release, brightening the skin, getting rid of dark circles under the eyes, and diminishing fine lines and wrinkles.

Chinese dermatologist Song Ping, M.D. notes that while Botox® injections and laser treatments are popular there, ingesting collagen protein, plus injecting collagen, are also popular among Chinese women for younger-looking skin.[116]

It's not surprising that many spas and beauty resorts in North America and Europe are incorporating ancient Asian beauty treatments into their spa menus today, too. With the interrelated and dynamic energies Mother Nature shares with

---

[116] Email received on 2/19/2011.

her mineral, plant, animal, and human kingdoms, it's only reasonable for people and environment to benefit from healing synergistically together—and in looking naturally beautiful, radiant, and glowing healthily—thanks to ancient herbal and healing medicinal practices that have proved their worth over centuries of use.

What are Some Unconventional Treatments?

Vanity and beauty are truly in the eye of those who would go under the knife to enhance their appearances for reasons ranging from getting ahead economically and socially at work to looking good. What are some unconventional treatments, and have they gone too far? Below are some examples.

1. <u>Ear, eye and nose jobs.</u> The *New York Times* reports an unusual procedure performed by Dr. Steve Lee, a plastic surgeon in Flushing, New York.[117] Apparently, the Chinese believe prominent earlobes invite, and are a sign of, wealth and prosperity. So, a gentleman had Dr. Lee inject a filler into his earlobes to extend them.

    Dr. Lee also has Chinese patients requesting their upturned noses be turned all the way down because of a traditional belief that prominent nostrils allow good fortune to spill out.

    Additionally, this article published on 2/19/2011 reports that in New York City, as well as in the Far East, double eyelid surgery is the most sought-after surgery among Asians.

2. <u>Bone lengthening.</u> In China, a controversial operation increases a person's height by breaking the

---

[117]

http://www.nytimes.com/2011/02/19/nyregion/19plastic.html?pagewanted=2&_r=2

leg bone to insert a metal lengthener. Pathetically, a *Marie Claire* magazine article reports, "For Chinese women, the pressure to be tall invades all aspects of life. Chinese society equates height with beauty and power."[118] This article compares leg lengthening to foot binding as a "taboo subject" that's rarely discussed. The mother of one patient told writer Brian Jones, "This is our secret. We're not going to advertise it. It will help with her future. We will be able to pay back the money when she gets a better job. She's very clever, and this will make all the difference." Sometimes, economic necessity can dictate less than prudent means when striving for personal and professional goals.

It's also quite a turnaround from ancient times when bound feet were the norm for petite Chinese women—compared to today's requirements of height for beauty, power, and employment prospects!

Let's conclude on a positive note in recognizing the legacy of an enduring beauty and healing regimen such as TCM. China's Herborist cosmetics website has a free "tai chi massage" tutorial that's downloadable. It shows how to rebalance energies of the upper yang section with the lower yin section of the face.[119] These "tai chi massage" techniques are similar to calming strokes aestheticians use for facials in western-style spas and beauty salons. In the U.S., Herborist products are only available at Sephora stores.

---

[118] http://www.east-asian-history.net/textbooks/PM-China/graphics/Ch11/25.htm
[119] http://www.herborist-international.com/wp-content/uploads/massage_tai_chi_UK.pdf

CHAPTER EIGHT

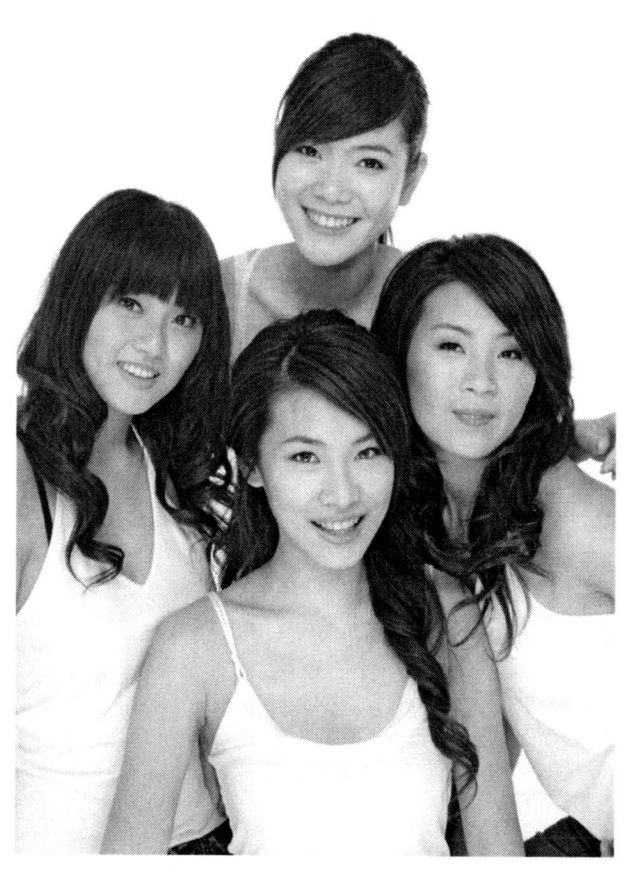

CHAPTER

8

Conclusion

One of the most significant differences between modern cosmetics and traditional Chinese medicine is that traditional Chinese medicine tries to achieve beauty by improving natural health.

Health is the most important factor for beauty, and natural beauty is a sign of a healthy body. In many cases, cosmetic problems are related to health problems.

As shown in this book, all of the ancient cosmetic formulas are to remove pathological factors and improve natural health, no matter whether the formula is for hair loss or for anti-wrinkle. Many of the formulas are also anti-aging recipes. While the formulas can be used to help one become more beautiful, they may also make one healthier and feel better. This is probably the ideal state of real health and beauty.
—Qing Yan, M.D., Ph.D. Author of *Herbs for Beauty: Imperial and Secret Herbal Formulas from Ancient China*
(PharmTao, 2005)

WE HAVE COVERED A wide range of ancient Asian beauty secrets and modern beauty treatments and techniques in the previous chapters. I hope you are inspired to try some of these ideas for your beauty resolutions and daily regimens. As Dr. Qing Yan points out, real beauty is radiant beauty—and glowing beauty is the true reflection of inner health. Outer beauty reflects good health that needs daily nurturing. Skin care is an important component of nurturing good health for joyful living and peace of mind in presenting a confident look, anytime.

CONCLUSIONS

From Korea:

- Centuries old herbal and healing medicines are helping modern cosmetics companies develop cutting-edge anti-aging skin care creams, such as Amore Pacific's Sulwhasoo Concentrated Ginger Cream and their other top-selling line—Moisture Bound Rejuvenating Crème formulated with deeply hydrating "divine water" or bamboo sap. Bamboo sap is also rich in antioxidants. Both qualities (deeply moisturizing and antioxidant-rich) have been, and are, enjoyed by Korean women in regenerating skin for a fresher, more youthful look. The results? Improved brightness and radiance, firmer skin, and a reduction in the appearance of wrinkles. Coupled with advanced nano-technology, these creams penetrate the skin effortlessly without clogging pores.

- Korea is also at the forefront of electronic laser technology for skin rejuvenation. For example, MedEdge, Inc., a Los Angeles-based company, states on its website, www.mededge-inc.com/lutronic.htm, "Well, we had to travel all the way to Korea, but we are truly convinced we have found the best available solution to the symptoms of melasma with the Lutronic USA line of medical and aesthetic lasers. Aesthetic practitioners throughout Asia and Europe have been achieving outstanding results with their melasma patients."[120]

---

[120] http://www.mededge-inc.com/lutronic.htm

It's also worth noting that Korean scientists have smartly combined the principles of acupuncture with dermal heating in coming up with intracel laser treatments based on FRM or "Fractional Radiofrequency Microneedling," mentioned in Chapter 7.[121] FRM is effective in tightening skin, reducing wrinkles, and erasing scars.

From Japan:

- Japanese beauty aesthetics are returning to tried and true secrets that are nature-based. From the healing facials of nightingales to seaweeds, black and red beans, and eating seasonally and locally, it's a healthy return to nature's pharmacy in looking good—with natural products.

- Japanese culture also recognizes the importance of rebalancing daily living with peaceful serenity—by engaging in meditative practices, such as the tea ceremony, meditating on nature, and making time for quiet time.

From China:

- Traditional Chinese Medicine (TCM) has been healing and promoting beautiful living for longevity and well-being for over 5,000 years. The efficacy of TCM continues today with Western medical practitioners integrating acupuncture, acupressure, and herbal medicines into their practices. Two notable resources for this book are: Jill Blakeway, the founder of New York City's YinOva Center, and Dr. Barbara Custer in Mill Valley, California.

---

[121] http://intracel.blogspot.com/

CONCLUSION

Most enduring of all are three common threads linking Korean, Japanese, and Chinese medical wisdom in promoting good health for beauty:

- Nature-based healing by prevailing on the plant and animal kingdoms for herbal concoctions.

- Food-based for nutritious healing that also promotes culinary enjoyment.

- Energy-based in rebalancing the body's vital force (qi), blood, and lymph so internal harmony promotes good health—and is reflected on the face and skin.

All three are products courtesy of Mother Nature and a testament to the efficacy of natural healing for beauty and lifelong well-being.

> *To live in the beauty*
> *And fragrance of the heart*
> *Is to get younger*
> *By the second.*
>
> —Sri Chinmoy, Meditation Master

BIBLIOGRAPHY

Gao, Duo, Dr., Editor. *The Encyclopedia of Chinese Medicine.* Carlton Books.1997.

Pitchford, Paul. *Healing with Whole Foods.* (3rd. edition) North Atlantic Books. 2002.

Saeki, Chizu. *The Japanese Skincare Revolution: How to Have the Most Beautiful Skin of Your Life—at Any Age.* Kodansha International. 2009.

Yan, Qing, M.D., Ph.D. *Herbs for Beauty: Imperial and Secret Herbal Formulas from Ancient China.* PharmTao. 2005.

ACKNOWLEDGEMENTS:

I am very grateful to my professional colleagues and friends for their help with ideas, references, and citations:

1) Jill Blakeway, M.S., L. Ac., Founder & Director, YinOva Center, New York City; www.yinovacenter.com

2) Dr. Hyung-Gi Cha, Dermatologist; Dreamfeel Dermatology Clinic, Kyonggi, South Korea

3) Dr. Gwang Seong Choi, M.D., Ph.D.; Professor and Chairman, Dept of Dermatology Inha University College, Seoul, South Korea

4) Dr. Barbara Custer, L. Ac., O.M.D.; Mill Valley, California; www.drbarbaracuster.com

5) Dr. Hyeonsook Lee, Dermatologist; Beauty & Clear Clinic, Seoul, South Korea; www.vipskin.co.kr

6) Dr. Song Ping, Associate Professor, Dept. of Dermatology, GuanAn'men Hospital, China Academy of Chinese Medical Services; Beijing

7) Mary Schook, "Beauty Engineer", New York City; www.maryschook.com

8) Ms. Liza Dalby, Anthropologist & Author (*Geisha*, etc.); www.lizadalby.com

9) Ms. Alice Lee, Senior Beauty Editor, Beijing Raylie Magazine House

10) Ms. Huang Ti, Deputy Beauty Editor, *Cosmo China*

11) Ms. Linda Huynh, Medical Assistant, Premier Dermatology, San Francisco & San Carlos, California; www.premier-dermatology.com

12) Ms. Yumi Kim, Owner, Curtain Call, Inc.; New York City; www.curtain-call.biz

13) Ms. Janice Mirikitani; Poet Laureate of San Francisco, Executive Director of Glide Church & President of Glide Foundation

14) Janelle Wang, TV Broadcaster, San Francisco

15) Jeremy Cheung, Shanghai and Seoul, www.justbb.com

16) Amy Chu, Princeton, NJ

17) Kimberley Davis, SF, CA

18) Ericka Erickson, Palo Alto, CA

19) Pepperann Huo, Singapore

20) Susan Kim, NYC

21) June Kwon, SF, CA

22) Jiyeon Kim, Seoul, South Korea

23) Grace Niwa, Boston, MA

24) Vera Sung, NYC

25) Naoko Tani-Fukuchi, Tokyo, Japan

26) Alison Diboll, SF, CA

27) Min Kim-Lee, Korean actress, Los Angeles, CA

28) Yuan Ting, Chinese actress, China

I would like to also thank the following people for all their support, encouragement, and belief in me:

Alicia Dunams

Sunamita Lim

My Premier Dermatology staff

My EO forum mates

Joyce's lunch group

My sisters: Anne, Jaclyn, and Joann

My mentors: Dr. Ken Lee, Dr. Michael Fisher, Dr. Marc Jacobson, Dr. Steven Cohen, Dr. Mike Eidelman, Dr. Jeanne Leddon, Dr. Roy Kim, Andy Cunningham

My girlfriends: Adriana, Anne, Stacie, Jean, Janet, Judy, Sara, Elinor, Nancy, Kimberley, June

My nannies: Suzy Seoung Lee and Jennifer Williams

ABOUT THE AUTHOR

D R. MARIE JHIN was born in Seoul, South Korea, and is a graduate of Wellesley College and Cornell University Medical College. A board certified dermatologist, Dr. Jhin is an Asian skin expert and director of Premier Dermatology in the San Francisco Bay area. She has been featured in numerous magazines, TV, newspapers and the Internet. She is a fellow of the American Academy of Dermatology, American Society for Dermatologic Surgery, and a member of the Women's Dermatologic Society. She has been rated as America's Top Doctor for the past three years. She was an Adjunct Clinical Instructor of Dermatology at Stanford University from 2001 to 2011.

To contact Dr. Marie Jhin, please visit:

Drmariejhin.com

9 780615 405353